Glycemic Control in the Hospitalized Patient

T0181742

Glycemic Control in the Hospitalized Patient

A Comprehensive Clinical Guide

Edited by

Lillian F. Lien, MD

Medical Director, Duke Inpatient Diabetes Management,
Department of Medicine, Division of Endocrinology, Metabolism, and Nutrition,
Duke University Medical Center, Durham, North Carolina

Mary E. Cox, MD, MHS

Department of Medicine, Division of Endocrinology, Metabolism, and Nutrition,
Duke University Medical Center, Durham, North Carolina

Mark N. Feinglos, MD, CM

Professor of Medicine, Chief, Division of Endocrinology, Metabolism,
and Nutrition, Duke University Medical Center, Durham, North Carolina

Leonor Corsino, MD, MHS

Instructor of Medicine, Department of Medicine, Division of Endocrinology,
Metabolism, and Nutrition, Duke University Medical Center, Durham,
North Carolina

Foreword by

Guillermo Umpierrez, MD, FACP, FACE

Professor of Medicine, Emory University School of Medicine

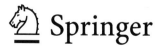 Springer

Editors
Lillian F. Lien, MD
Division of Endocrinology,
 Metabolism, and Nutrition
Department of Medicine
Duke University Medical Center Box 2956
Durham, NC 27710, USA
lien0002@mc.duke.edu

Mary E. Cox, MD, MHS
Division of Endocrinology,
 Metabolism, and Nutrition
Department of Medicine
Duke University Medical Center
Durham, NC 27710, USA
marybethcoxmd@gmail.com

Mark N. Feinglos, MD, CM
Division of Endocrinology,
 Metabolism, and Nutrition
Department of Medicine
Duke University Medical Center
Baker House Trent Drive
Durham, NC 27710, USA
feing002@mc.duke.edu

Leonor Corsino, MD, MHS
Division of Endocrinology,
 Metabolism, and Nutrition
Department of Medicine
Duke University Medical Center Box 3921
Durham, NC 27710, USA
corsi002@mc.duke.edu

ISBN 978-1-60761-005-2   e-ISBN 978-1-60761-006-9
DOI 10.1007/978-1-60761-006-9
Springer New York Dordrecht Heidelberg London

Library of Congress Control Number: 2010935296

© Springer Science+Business Media, LLC 2011
All rights reserved. This work may not be translated or copied in whole or in part without the written permission of the publisher (Springer Science+Business Media, LLC, 233 Spring Street, New York, NY 10013, USA), except for brief excerpts in connection with reviews or scholarly analysis. Use in connection with any form of information storage and retrieval, electronic adaptation, computer software, or by similar or dissimilar methodology now known or hereafter developed is forbidden.
The use in this publication of trade names, trademarks, service marks, and similar terms, even if they are not identified as such, is not to be taken as an expression of opinion as to whether or not they are subject to proprietary rights.
While the advice and information in this book are believed to be true and accurate at the date of going to press, neither the authors nor the editors nor the publisher can accept any legal responsibility for any errors or omissions that may be made. The publisher makes no warranty, express or implied, with respect to the material contained herein.

Printed on acid-free paper

Springer is part of Springer Science+Business Media (www.springer.com)

Disclaimer

The views expressed in this book are those of the authors and do not necessarily represent the views of Duke University and the Durham Veterans Affairs Medical Center.

This book contains information intended as an educational aid. This book is not intended as medical advice for individual patients or conditions. The suggestions in this book do not substitute for a medical exam and do not replace the need for evaluation and judgment of medical professionals. Although the authors have done their best to ensure full integrity of the work, the publisher, editors, and authors do not assume any risk for the use of suggestions contained within this book. Please inform us of any inaccuracies so they may be corrected in future editions.

To my mom and dad, Mei-fong W. Lien and Stephen Lien, for love and great wisdom: you are my inspiration. In loving memory of Sheue Lin Wang.

-Lillian F. Lien, MD

To my husband, Bryan, and to Mom and Dad, for your love and support.

-Mary E. Cox, MD MHS

To my mother and husband, Luz Maria and Carlos, for their unconditional support; in memory of my father, Damian, who battled diabetes for over 30 years.

-Leonor Corsino, MD MHS

Foreword

I am pleased to write the foreword for the first edition of this book entitled Glycemic Control in the Hospitalized Patient. The text is written by a group of expert healthcare providers at Duke University Medical Center who have extensive experience in the management of hospitalized individuals with hyperglycemia. The experience of the authors is highly valuable as they come from an institution that was one of the earliest to develop an inpatient Diabetes Management Service. In this book, the reader will find detailed and focused guidance for the management of hyperglycemia and hypoglycemia in situations which are unique to the inpatient setting, such as enteral and parenteral nutrition, intravenous insulin, and insulin pumps. This book should be useful for providers at all levels, from medical students, to interns and residents, and our endocrine fellows and other colleagues. I believe that the reader will find this text useful in achieving the ultimate goal of providing high quality care for all patients in the hospital.

Atlanta, GA   Guillermo Umpierrez

Preface

Rationale for Inpatient Management of Hyperglycemia

The number of people with diabetes mellitus continues to increase at an alarming rate. It is estimated that the number of individuals diagnosed with diabetes worldwide will be approximately 366 million by the year 2030. With this rapidly growing group of people diagnosed with diabetes, it is not surprising that the proportion of individuals admitted to the hospital with diabetes as a comorbidity is elevated as well. Additionally, a significant number of patients without a prior diagnosis of diabetes will develop hyperglycemia during hospitalization.

In recent years, there has been an evolution in the management of hospitalized patients with hyperglycemia. Inconsistent clinical trial results urged experts in the field to reconsider the targets of control warranted in hospitalized patients. However, despite some of the existent controversy generated by these clinical trial results, most experts agree that hyperglycemia in the hospitalized patient cannot be ignored and that appropriate management continues to be critical.

One of the major issues addressed during the controversy was the potential deleterious effect of tight glycemic control (80–110 mg/dL [4.4–6.1 mmol/L]) in both critically and noncritically ill patients and those at risk for hypoglycemia. Based on the fact that some of these studies failed to demonstrate significant improvement in mortality in the intensive care unit patient and some showed a possible increase, it is clear that the controversy continues and glycemic targets should be reconsidered in order to avoid potential patient harm. However, it is our hope, and the hope of many experts in the field, that patients admitted to the hospital with a history of diabetes and those with newly developed hyperglycemia will be carefully monitored and treated.

The most recent consensus statement on this topic from the American Diabetes Association and the American Association of Clinical Endocrinologists addressed the current evidence both against and in favor of glycemic control in hospitalized patients and recommended that therapy should be initiated in critically ill patients with persistent hyperglycemia, starting with a threshold of no greater than 180 mg/dL (10 mmol/L) and, once insulin is started, therapy should target a glucose range of 140–180 mg/dL (7.8–10 mmol/L). For noncritically ill patients, the glucose target should generally be a fasting glucose of less than 140 mg/dL (7.8 mmol/L) and random glucose of less than 180 mg/dL (10 mmol/L), providing that these goals can be achieved safely.

The goal of this book is to provide a very useful and practical resource for healthcare providers who treat hyperglycemia in the inpatient setting. The authors have included a practical approach to different scenarios that occur while treating patients with hyperglycemia, such as patients receiving enteral nutrition. Additionally, the book serves as a comprehensive guide to all aspects of inpatient glycemic control, such as the initiation of insulin, treatment of hypoglycemia, and the transition of care to the outpatient setting. The ultimate goal of the contributors is to improve the quality of care and quality of life of our patients with diabetes and those with hyperglycemia in the inpatient setting.

Finally, the editors would like to acknowledge Dr Corsino for her idea of writing a book that provides guidance to healthcare providers taking care of patients with hyperglycemia in the inpatient setting and for making this book a reality. In addition, the editors would like to thank our contributors for their hard work and for their continued efforts to improve the care of patients with diabetes.

Durham, NC   Lillian F. Lien
                                                                                       Mary E. Cox
                                                                                   Mark N. Feinglos
                                                                                   Leonor Corsino

Special Acknowledgments

We wish to give special thanks to the following individuals, who provided particular assistance to the editors and authors in the preparation of this book:

From our publishers, we especially thank Richard Lansing for his assistance and for believing in our project, as well as Robin Weisberg, style editor, for her excellent work.

From Duke University Medical Center, we thank Mary Jane Stillwagon and the Duke Hospital Glycemic Safety Committee, as well as Melanie Mabrey, Sarah Gauger, Ellen Davis, Daniel Feinglos, and Mark Feinglos for expertise and friendship.

We also wish to acknowledge individuals from Abbott, Michelle L Zendah and Linda A Murray, as well as Nestle, Marilyn Cook and Sally Crush, who assisted us with permissions to use their material.

Finally, we thank our colleagues and patients for their insights and strength.

Contents

1   **Physiology of Diabetes Mellitus and Types of Insulin**   1
    Bryan C. Batch, Mary E. Cox, and Lillian F. Lien

2   **Subcutaneous Insulin: A Guide for Dosing Regimens
    in the Hospital**   7
    Karen Barnard, Bryan C. Batch, and Lillian F. Lien

3   **IV Insulin Infusions: How to Use an "Insulin Drip"**   17
    Melanie E. Mabrey and Lillian F. Lien

4   **Laboratory Testing in Hospitalized Patients
    with Diabetes Mellitus**   29
    Karen Barnard and Mary E. Cox

5   **Inpatient Diabetes Education: Realistic and Evidence-Based**   41
    Ellen D. Davis, Anne T. Nettles, and Ashley Leak

6   **Hyperglycemic Emergencies: Diabetic Ketoacidosis
    and Hyperosmolar Hyperglycemic State**   51
    Leonor Corsino and Lekshmi T. Nair

7   **Medical Nutrition Therapy in the Hospital**   63
    Sarah Gauger

8   **Insulin Pumps and Glucose Sensors in the Hospital**   67
    Sarah Gauger

9   **Non-insulin Antidiabetic Medications
    in the Inpatient Setting**   77
    Jennifer V. Rowell, Lekshmi T. Nair, and Mary E. Cox

10 **Hypoglycemia**   91
    Melanie E. Mabrey, Mary E. Cox, and Lillian F. Lien

11 **Transitioning to Outpatient Care**   101
    Beatrice D. Hong and Ellen D. Davis

12   **Management of Hyperglycemia Associated with Enteral
     and Parenteral Nutrition**   113
     Sarah Gauger

13   **When to Consult Endocrinology**   119
     Beatrice D. Hong

14   **Frequently Asked Questions**   121
     Mary E. Cox and Matthew J. Crowley

Subject Index   139

Contributors

Karen Barnard Division of Endocrinology, Metabolism, and Nutrition, Department of Medicine, Duke University Medical Center, Durham, NC 27710, USA; Department of Veterans Affairs, Durham, NC 27707, USA, karen.barnard@duke.edu

Bryan C. Batch Division of Endocrinology, Metabolism, and Nutrition, Department of Medicine, Duke University Medical Center, Durham, NC 27710, USA; Department of Veterans Affairs, Durham, NC 27707, USA, bryan.batch@duke.edu

Leonor Corsino Division of Endocrinology, Metabolism, and Nutrition, Department of Medicine, Duke University Medical Center, Durham, NC 27710, USA, corsi002@mc.duke.edu

Mary E. Cox Division of Endocrinology, Metabolism, and Nutrition, Department of Medicine, Duke University Medical Center, Durham, NC 27710, USA, marybethcoxmd@gmail.com

Matthew J. Crowley Division of Endocrinology, Metabolism, and Nutrition, Department of Medicine, Duke University Medical Center, Durham, NC 27710, USA, matthew.crowley@duke.edu

Ellen D. Davis Department of Advanced Clinical Practice, Duke University Hospital, Durham, NC 27710, USA; Duke University School of Nursing, Durham, NC 27710, USA, davis010@mc.duke.edu

Sarah Gauger Duke Inpatient Diabetes Management, Duke University Medical Center, Durham, NC 27710, USA, gauge003@mc.duke.edu

Beatrice D. Hong Division of Endocrinology, Metabolism and Nutrition, Department of Medicine, Duke University Medical Center, Durham, NC 27710, USA, beatrice.hong@duke.edu

Ashley Leak Accelerated BSN Program, Duke University School of Nursing, John A. Hartford Building Academic Geriatric Nursing Capacity (BAGNC)

Scholar, 2009–2011, Durham, NC, USA; UNC-Chapel Hill School of Nursing, Durham, NC, USA, ashley.leak@duke.edu

Lillian F. Lien Division of Endocrinology, Metabolism, and Nutrition, Department of Medicine, Durham, NC 27710, USA; Duke Inpatient Diabetes Management, Duke University Medical Center, Durham, NC 27710, USA, lien0002@mc.duke.edu

Melanie E. Mabrey Duke Inpatient Diabetes Management, Department of Advanced Clinical Practice, Duke University Hospital, Durham, NC, USA; Duke University Schools of Nursing and Medicine, Duke University Medical Center, Durham, NC, USA, mabre002@mc.duke.edu

Lekshmi T. Nair Division of Endocrinology, Metabolism, and Nutrition, Department of Medicine, Duke University Medical Center, Durham, NC 27710, USA, ltnair@gmail.com

Anne T. Nettles Diabetes CareWorks, Wayzata, MN, USA, anne@diabetescareworks.com

Jennifer V. Rowell Division of Endocrinology, Metabolism, and Nutrition, Department of Medicine, Duke University Medical Center, Durham, NC 27710, USA, jennifer.rowell@duke.edu

Chapter 1
Physiology of Diabetes Mellitus and Types of Insulin

Bryan C. Batch, Mary E. Cox, and Lillian F. Lien

Keywords Type 1 diabetes · Type 2 diabetes · MODY · Insulin resistance · Aspart insulin (Novolog®) · Lispro insulin (Humalog®) · Glulisine insulin (Apidra®) · Regular insulin (Humulin® · Novolin®) · NPH insulin · Detemir insulin (Levemir®) · Glargine insulin (Lantus®)

Prevalence

In 2008, the Centers for Disease Control and Prevention (CDC) estimated that 24 million people in the United States had diabetes mellitus, constituting nearly 8% of the population. The CDC further estimated that 57 million individuals were affected by prediabetes, and approximately 10% of those with prediabetes will progress to diabetes each year. Because of this large population of individuals who now have and who will have diabetes in the near future, it is important for providers to have a basic understanding of diabetes pathophysiology and to thoughtfully pursue appropriate diagnoses.

The American Diabetes Association (ADA) has defined diagnostic criteria for diabetes and prediabetes (Table 1.1).

Pathophysiology

Glucose homeostasis is a balance of many factors, including insulin release from the pancreas, central and peripheral insulin utilization, and endogenous production and exogenous intake of glucose. Both insulin release and insulin utilization are, in turn, modulated by many cytokines and hormones. When either insulin release is insufficient or insulin utilization is incomplete (i.e., insulin resistance), diabetes mellitus is the result.

B.C. Batch (✉)
Division of Endocrinology, Metabolism, and Nutrition, Department of Medicine, Duke University Medical Center, Durham, NC 27710, USA; Department of Veterans Affairs, Durham, NC 27707, USA
e-mail: bryan.batch@duke.edu

L.F. Lien et al. (eds.), *Glycemic Control in the Hospitalized Patient*,
DOI 10.1007/978-1-60761-006-9_1, © Springer Science+Business Media, LLC 2011

Table 1.1 American Diabetes Association diagnostic criteria for prediabetes and diabetes

Diagnosis	Diagnostic test
Prediabetes: impaired fasting glucose[a]	Fasting plasma glucose of 100–125 mg/dL (5.5–6.9 mmol/L)
Prediabetes: impaired glucose tolerance[a]	75-g OGTT 2-h plasma glucose of 140–199 mg/dL (7.7–11 mmol/L)
Diabetes	Fasting plasma glucose ≥126 mg/dL (7 mmol/L)
	Or
	Random plasma glucose ≥200 mg/dL (≥11.1 mmol/L) with symptoms of diabetes (polyuria, polydipsia, unexplained weight loss)
	Or
	75-g OGTT 2-h plasma glucose ≥200 mg/dL (≥ 11.1 mmol/L)
	Or
	A_{1c} ≥6.5%

OGTT, oral glucose tolerance test
[a]There is no formal A_{1C} cut-off point that defines the category of prediabetes, but values between 5.7 and 6.5% suggest patients who are "at risk"

There are two main forms of diabetes, types 1 and 2 (Table 1.2). Although the clinical results of hyperglycemia and related complications are similar among the types of diabetes, establishment of a clinical distinction is important to guide appropriate management. This being said, it is important to recognize that it may not always be possible to classify patients firmly as having "either" type 1 or type 2,

Table 1.2 Characteristics of type 1 and type 2 diabetes[a]

Characteristic	Type 1 diabetes	Type 2 diabetes
Age at onset	Young; typically <40 years of age	Adult
Symptoms at diagnosis	Polyuria, polydipsia, weight loss; patients typically are ill at the time of presentation	May be detected on routine screening or present with symptoms
Cause of diabetes	Pancreatic destruction	Insulin resistance in combination with β-cell dysfunction
Weight	Normal	Overweight or obese
Family history	~10%	>90%
Presence of antibodies	Present in 90%	Uncommon
Acute complications	DKA	Hyperosmolar nonketotic hyperglycemia; DKA is rare
C-peptide or endogenous insulin level	Low	Normal or high

DKA, diabetic ketoacidosis
[a]For each characteristic of disease, there may be exceptions. The distinction between type 1 and type 2 diabetes must be made based on a compilation of all of the clinical evidence rather than with any single characteristic

given the reality that diabetes mellitus actually encompasses a group of heterogeneous disorders. Here, we discuss the basic underlying pathophysiology and clinical characteristics of the two major types of diabetes, as well as a hereditary form of diabetes called maturity onset diabetes of the young (MODY).

Type 1 Diabetes

Type 1 diabetes presents with an absolute deficit of pancreatic insulin production due to T cell-mediated destruction of the β-cells. Additionally, autoantibodies have been detected in up to 90% of patients with immune-mediated diabetes. The stimulus for this autoimmune destruction is not well understood. Type 1 diabetes results in an absolute insulin deficiency and must be treated with exogenous insulin.

Individuals with type 1 diabetes often are affected from a young age, although there is a subset of patients who present with immune-mediated diabetes at an older age. This is called latent autoimmune diabetes of the adult (LADA). All patients with type 1 diabetes are at risk for the acute complication of diabetic ketoacidosis, as described in Chapter 6. Other characteristics of the disease can be seen in Table 1.2.

Diseases that result in destruction of the pancreas from nonimmune causes, such as pancreatectomy, pancreatitis, and cystic fibrosis, will result in a similar insulin deficiency and require treatment with insulin. Many of these patients have additional problems with glucose homeostasis and will require management by an endocrinologist.

Type 2 Diabetes

Type 2 diabetes has a complex physiology involving many processes that, together, lead to hyperglycemia and its associated complications. Individuals with type 2 diabetes often are overweight or obese, and caloric excess is a key precipitant. This contributes to excess adiposity and insulin resistance. However, adiposity and peripheral insulin resistance are not the only factors; β-cell dysfunction appears to play a pivotal role as well. Prevention and treatment of type 2 diabetes must be directed at both pathologic components: preservation of β-cell function and improvement in insulin resistance. This therapy leans heavily toward lifestyle modification via healthy eating and exercise, and it comes to incorporate many types of medical therapies as well.

MODY

MODY is an uncommon, autosomal dominant form of diabetes, sometimes referred to as "monogenic" diabetes. There are various forms of MODY, which vary in severity from manageable with diet to completely dependent on insulin. The pathologic deficit is at the level of insulin secretion, although some amount of insulin secretion often is maintained. It is important to distinguish MODY from other types of diabetes, as the hyperglycemia in patients with MODY often responds very well to sulfonylurea medications. Individuals who are suspected to have MODY should be referred to an endocrinologist for assessment and counseling.

Types of Exogenous Insulin

The most common treatment for hyperglycemia in the inpatient setting is the administration of subcutaneous insulin. The insulin formulations available today far exceed what was available even a decade ago. Although this variety of formulations enables providers to individualize therapy for each patient's unique needs, it also creates opportunity for confusion. Inpatient providers must be attentive to details of their patients' regimens to avoid medication errors. The insulins are categorized according to their durations of action: rapid-, short-, intermediate-, and long-acting (Table 1.3).

Table 1.3 Types of insulin

Insulin type	Lispro (Humalog®) Aspart (Novolog®) Glulisine (Apidra®)	Regular (Humulin®, Novolin®)	NPH	Glargine (Lantus®)	Detemir (Levemir®)
Onset of action	15–30 min rapid-acting	30 min short-acting	1–2 h intermediate-acting	1–2 h long-acting	~1 h long-acting
Time to peak	1–2 h	2–4 h	4–10 h	No peak	No/little peak
Duration	3–5 h	4–8 h (subcutaneous)	12–20 h	~24 h	Up to 24 h
Administration	≤15 min before meals or immediately after meals	30–60 min before meals	30–60 min before meals or at bedtime	Without regard to meals; usually at bedtime	Without regard to meals; daily to twice per day

Rapid-Acting Insulin: Lispro (Humalog®), Aspart (Novolog®), and Glulisine (Apidra®)

The rapid-acting insulin formulations, also called analog insulins, are characterized by a rapid onset (15–30 min), rapid peak (1–2 h), and limited duration (3–5 h). Because of the rapid onset of action, these insulin formulations must be accompanied by food. Specifically, they should be administered no more than 15 min prior to meals or, in the case of uncertain food intake, they can be given immediately after meals. If a patient is temporarily fasting, then the rapid-acting insulin should not be given.

Short-Acting Insulin: Regular (Novolin®, Humulin®)

Like the rapid-acting insulins, regular insulin typically is given for prandial coverage. A basal-prandial insulin regimen containing regular insulin usually consists of regular insulin injected with each meal (breakfast, lunch, and supper), accompanied by an injection of neutral protamine hagedorn (NPH) insulin at bedtime.

Regular insulin must be given 30 min before meals and can be expected to reach its peak activity approximately 2–4 h later. Its duration of action lasts 4–8 h. Regular insulin has the advantage of being inexpensive, and it can be mixed in a syringe with NPH insulin if patients require concomitant administration. However, some patients and providers find that it is inconvenient to administer insulin 30 min prior to mealtime. Additionally, use of regular insulin leads to a slightly greater risk for hypoglycemia than use of the newer insulin analogs. For these reasons, some providers are moving away from its use for prandial coverage.

Intermediate-Acting Insulin: Neutral Protamine Hagedorn

NPH insulin is considered an intermediate-acting insulin, with a prolonged duration of action over 12–20 h. It has an onset of action time of 1–2 h, and a peak action time of 4–10 h. NPH insulin commonly is given for basal coverage, either at bedtime, in the morning, or at both times. It also can be combined with regular insulin for a mixed preparation. Like regular insulin, NPH insulin is fairly inexpensive, and it can be mixed with regular insulin. The disadvantage of NPH insulin is that its delayed peak may cause hypoglycemia. For this reason, some providers prefer to replace NPH with one of the newer long-acting insulins.

Mixture of Regular and NPH Insulin

This combination typically is not recommended in the hospital and should be continued only if the patient is stable on this regimen at home and when other factors, such as diet, activity level, and scheduled procedures, have been considered. When mixing regular and NPH insulin, the regular insulin must be drawn into the syringe first, so that contamination of the regular insulin with NPH insulin will not occur. This contamination could alter the kinetics of the regular insulin. There are a variety of available premixed insulin formulations (Table 1.4), but we do not recommend their routine use in the hospital.

Table 1.4 Premixed insulin formulations

Combination insulins	Long-acting component	Short-acting component
Humulin® 70/30™ or Novolin® 70/30™	70% NPH	30% regular
NovoLog Mix® 70/30™	70% aspart-protamine suspension	30% aspart
Humalog Mix® 75/25™	75% lispro-protamine suspension	25% lispro

Long-Acting (Basal) Insulin: Glargine (Lantus®) and Detemir (Levemir®)

Glargine and detemir insulins are unique basal insulin formulations that have little to no true peak. Their duration of action is up to 24 h. These insulins have the advantage of provision of "smooth" basal coverage, reducing the risk for hypoglycemia that can be seen with insulins that peak. However, some patients will experience a peak effect with these formulations, and glucoses should be monitored regularly as with use of all insulins. It should be noted that long-acting insulins cannot be mixed in a syringe with other insulins.

For more information on how to properly dose and administer the various insulins discussed above, see Chapter 2: Subcutaneous Insulin and Chapter 11: Transition to Outpatient Care.

Bibliography

American Diabetes Association. Multiple-component insulin regimens. In: Farkas-Hirsch R, ed. *Intensive Diabetes Management*. Alexandria, VA: ADA, Inc; 1995:51–64.

American Diabetes Association: Executive Summary from the American Diabetes Association. Standards of medical care in Diabetes 2009. *Diabetes Care*. 2009; 32(suppl 1): S6–S12.

Diabetes Control and Complications Trial Research Group. The effect of intensive treatment of diabetes on the development and progression of long-term complications in insulin-dependent diabetes mellitus. *N Engl J Med*. 1993; 329(14):977–986.

Expert Committee on the Diagnosis and Classification of Diabetes Mellitus. *Diabetes Care*. 1998;21(suppl 1): S5–S19.

Henderson KE, Baranski TJ, Bickel PE, Clutter WE, McGill JB, eds. *The Washington Manual Endocrinology Subspecialty Consult*. 2nd ed. Philadelphia, PA: Lippincott Williams & Wilkins; 2009.

Leahy JL. Pathogenesis of type 2 diabetes mellitus. In: Feinglos MN, Bethel MA, eds. *Type 2 Diabetes Mellitus: An Evidence-Based Approach to Practical Management*. Totowa, NJ: Humana Press; 2008:17–33.

Lien LF, Bethel MA, Feinglos MN. In-hospital management of type 2 diabetes mellitus. *Med Clin N Am*. 2004; 88(4):1085–1105.

Muoio D, Newgard C. Molecular and metabolic mechanisms of insulin resistance and β-cell failure in type 2 diabetes. *Nat Rev Mol Cell Biol*. 2008; 9(3):193–205.

Nathan D. Insulin treatment of type 2 diabetes mellitus. In: Prote D, Sherwin R, Baron A, eds. *Ellenberg and Rifkin's Diabetes Mellitus*. 6th ed. New York, NY: McGraw-Hill; 2003:515–522.

Nathan M, Leahy J. Insulin management of hospitalized diabetic patients. In: Leahy J, Cefalu W, eds. *Insulin Therapy*. New York, NY: Marcel Dekker, Inc; 2002:153–172.

Number of people with diabetes increases to 24 million: estimates of diagnosed diabetes now available for all US. counties [CDC Online Newsroom press release]. Atlanta, GA: CDC. http://www.cdc.gov/media/pressrel/2008/r080624.htm. Accessed December 1, 2009.

Pearce SH, Merriman TR. Genetics of type 1 diabetes and autoimmune thyroid disease. *Endocrinol Metab Clin North Am*. 2009; 38(2):289–301.

Pratley R. Islet dysfunction: an underlying defect in the pathophysiology of type 2 diabetes. *Endocrinol Metab Clin North Am*. 2006; 35(suppl 1):6–11.

Waldron-Lynch F, Herold KC. Advances in type 1 diabetes therapeutics: immunomodulation and beta-cell salvage. *Endocrinol Metab Clin North Am*. 2009; 38(2):303–317.

Wittlin S, Woehrle H, Gerich J. Insulin pharmacokinetics. In: Leahy J, Cefalu W, eds. *Insulin Therapy*. New York, NY: Marcel Dekker, Inc; 2002:73–85.

Chapter 2
Subcutaneous Insulin: A Guide for Dosing Regimens in the Hospital

Karen Barnard, Bryan C. Batch, and Lillian F. Lien

Keywords Basal-bolus insulin · Prandial insulin · Basal insulin · Correction dose insulin · Total daily dose of insulin

Basal-Bolus Insulin

Insulin continues to be the preferred method for the management of hyperglycemia in the inpatient setting. It can be titrated easily, does not have a ceiling dose, and can be administered intravenously and subcutaneously. Details of IV insulin, including the transition from IV to subcutaneous, are discussed in Chapter 3: IV Insulin. In this chapter, we focus on subcutaneous insulin regimens.

Many patients who require subcutaneous insulin in the hospital will already have a diagnosis of diabetes; some will have been on insulin prior to admission. However, some nondiabetic patients may develop hyperglycemia as well. For all inpatients with hyperglycemia, we recommend a proactive insulin regimen that includes two components: (1) basal insulin, to cover basal insulin needs (mainly due to hepatic glucose production) and (2) bolus (or prandial) insulin, to cover any forms of caloric intake—meals, enteral feedings, or total parenteral nutrition (TPN). This strategy is referred to as basal-bolus insulin. For patients with type 1 diabetes, the basal-bolus insulin strategy is optimal, and these patients should always receive basal insulin, even during periods of fasting. Patients with type 1 diabetes require exogenous insulin to prevent the production of ketones and the subsequent development of diabetic ketoacidosis (DKA). For patients with type 2 diabetes also, the basal-bolus insulin strategy is preferred; however, the insulin requirement may decrease over periods of prolonged fasting. Current evidence supports the basal-bolus regimen as more effective, easier to design and adjust, better for blood glucose control, and lower risk for hypoglycemia than alternative strategies.

K. Barnard (✉)
Department of Medicine, Division of Endocrinology, Metabolism, and Nutrition, Duke University Medical Center, Durham, NC 27710, USA
e-mail: karen.barnard@duke.edu

L.F. Lien et al. (eds.), *Glycemic Control in the Hospitalized Patient*,
DOI 10.1007/978-1-60761-006-9_2, © Springer Science+Business Media, LLC 2011

An optional insulin regimen component is the correctional insulin scale (so-called sliding scale). The scale is used before meals along with the bolus insulin to correct hyperglycemia. The correctional insulin scale should not be used alone for patients with diabetes; this reactive strategy will not be effective to prevent hyperglycemia or inpatient complications such as hypoglycemia.

Special Care Situations

Subcutaneous insulin may not always be appropriate for patients in the intensive care unit, particularly those with severe sepsis, requiring vasopressors, with acute hepatic failure, or with severe hypoalbuminemia. In these patients IV insulin may be a better choice. An endocrinology consultant can assist with decision making in situations such as these.

Key Points: Basal-Bolus Insulin

- Insulin strategy: Basal + bolus + correctional insulin scale (optimal insulin regimen)
- Correctional insulin scale: avoid using as only insulin regimen. It is only good for patients who are at risk for hyperglycemia, but who do not currently have hyperglycemia.
- Patients with type 1 diabetes always require basal insulin, even if they are not eating.

Transition from Outpatient to Inpatient Care

A patient's outpatient regimen may not be appropriate in the inpatient setting for a variety of reasons.
- Stress can either increase or decrease a patient's insulin requirements.
- Nutrition in the hospital may be different from that at home (i.e., carbohydrate content, total calories, periods of fasting, etc., may be different).
- Medical conditions, such as hypotension, vasopressor use, edema, acute renal failure, surgical procedures, may alter insulin requirements.
- The insulin dose at home may not have provided adequate control.
- For patients who use premixed (2 shots/day) insulin products, such as 70/30 (Humulin 70/30; Novolog® Mix 70/30) and 50/50 (Humulin 50/50; Humalog Mix 50/50) at home: These components are not easily titrated in the inpatient setting. We recommend transition to a basal-bolus insulin regimen while these patients are hospitalized.
- Patients who have no prior diagnosis of diabetes, but who are at risk for developing hyperglycemia in the hospital (such as those receiving glucocorticoids or other medications, or TPN or enteral nutrition [EN]), should have their glucose closely monitored. If a patient develops consistent hyperglycemia, scheduled basal-bolus insulin should be initiated.

Glucose Monitoring

How Often to Monitor?

The frequency of monitoring will depend on the patient's nutrition pattern and insulin regimen.

- Patients eating scheduled meals should be monitored before meals, at bedtime, and, for some, at 3 AM. The 3 AM level can aid in interpretation of an elevated fasting glucose; potential causes include the "dawn phenomenon" and the "Somogyi effect," a rebound rise in blood glucose after hypoglycemia. Once glucoses are stable overnight, the 3 AM check can be discontinued.
- Patients receiving enteral feeding in boluses should be monitored prior to each bolus while the insulin regimen is still being adjusted. Once the insulin dose is stable, monitoring every 6 h is usually sufficient.
- If a patient has symptoms that could be consistent with hyper- or hypoglycemia, the glucose should be checked immediately, even if it is not a prescribed monitoring time.

Blood Glucose Targets

Over the last several years, the optimal glycemic target for the hospitalized patient with hyperglycemia has been the focus of significant discussion and controversy. However, it is reasonable to pursue the following as a straightforward set of goals that can be used in the treatment of most inpatients:

- Pre-meal blood glucose less than 140 mg/dL (7.8 mmol/L)
- Random blood glucose of less than 180 mg/dL (10.0 mmol/L)
- Recent discussions of glycemic control have emphasized the importance of individualizing targets. The selection of a more or less stringent target will depend on the patient's history of previous glucose control and current medical status (e.g., less stringent in patients with terminal illness and those with history of hypoglycemia unawareness).

Choosing an Insulin Regimen

The calculations recommended in this chapter are estimates and are meant to be a starting point. Always use clinical judgment, and make adjustments based on glucose readings obtained over the subsequent 24 h.

Obtain Baseline Information

Subjective: Type of diabetes, new or established, home medications (insulin and non-insulin), total daily dose (TDD) of insulin at home, hypoglycemia frequency, and symptoms.

Objective: Age, weight, height, body mass index (BMI), previous hemoglobin A$_{1C}$ (if available), glomerular filtration rate (GFR), liver function tests, nutritional status in the hospital, use of new medications such as glucocorticoids.

Calculate the Total Daily Insulin Dose

General Considerations

As discussed earlier in this chapter, multiple factors can affect the insulin regimen of a hospitalized patient. Although the degree of glycemic control optimal for the hospitalized patient is still debated, there is no debate regarding the importance of avoiding hypoglycemia. Insulin dosages can be rapidly and easily titrated upward, so it is reasonable to start near the low end of an estimated dose calculation and to ensure that necessary adjustments are made promptly. For patients with GFR less than 60 (stage III or higher chronic kidney disease (CKD), as well as those with acute renal failure), see the section on renal impairment below.

- For patients with type 1 diabetes, the total daily insulin dosage can be estimated at 0.3–0.5 units/kg/day. Patients with type 1 diabetes often are quite sensitive to insulin; thus, it is reasonable to start on the low end.
- For patients with type 2 diabetes, the total daily insulin dosage can start at 0.3–0.7 units/kg/day. Patients with type 2 diabetes have varying degrees of insulin resistance, so a patient who is new to insulin, with uncertain needs, may benefit from a relatively low dose to start. However, some patients may require more than 1 unit/kg/day. If there is uncertainty about the level of insulin resistance, it is simple and safe to start with a TDD of 0.5 units/kg/day.

Scenarios and Examples

Scenario 1: Patient with Hyperglycemia (With or Without Diabetes) Who Is New to Insulin

The patient is new to insulin, so it is reasonable to start with a TDD of 0.3 units/kg/day. However, a higher TDD may be implemented in certain cases. 0.1 units/kg/day can be added to the TDD for the presence of each of the following:

- The patient has type 2 diabetes and is less than 70 years old.
- The patient has evidence of difficult control; that is, he or she takes at least three oral agents at home, or the hemoglobin A$_{1C}$ is greater than 8%, or he or she reports fasting glucoses greater than 200 mg/dL (11.0 mmol/L) prior to admission.
- The patient has a BMI greater than 35 kg/m^2.

For example, a 40-year-old patient with type 2 diabetes who has never used insulin, whose preadmission A$_{1C}$ is 9%, and whose BMI is 36 kg/m^2, could reasonably be given a TDD of 0.6 units/kg/day.

Scenario 2: Patient with Type 2 Diabetes, on Known Dosages of Insulin at Home

The first step is to determine the patient's true TDD. Consistency of usage is an important component of the history. Does the patient always take the prescribed dosage, or does he or she make modifications? How often does he or she miss an insulin dose?

In order to determine the safety of the patient's reported TDD, it is helpful to calculate a weight-adjusted TDD based on units per kilogram per day. For example, a patient has type 2 diabetes and normally takes 40 units of insulin per day. He weighs 80 kg. His weight-based TDD is 40 units/80 kg/day, or 0.5 units/kg/day. This is reasonable and likely to be safe for a patient with type 2 diabetes. Based on this calculation, it is reasonable to continue with the patient's home TDD in the hospital. If the dose seems too high, a smaller dose can be used initially, with prompt increases as deemed necessary from monitored glucose values.

A list of situations for which the insulin dose can be modified is found in Table 2.1.

Table 2.1 Situations warranting cautious modification of home total daily dose of insulin[a]

Situation	Modification
Type 1 diabetes and uncontrolled glucoses (A_{1C} >8%) or fasting glucoses >200 mg/dL (11 mmol/L)	↑home TDD by 10%
Type 2 diabetes and uncontrolled glucoses (A_{1C} >8%) or fasting glucoses >200 mg/dL (11 mmol/L)	↑ home TDD by 20%
Patient is ABOUT TO BEGIN corticosteroids (newly prescribed for the inpatient stay)	↑ home TDD by 20%
Patient reports hypoglycemia unawareness	↓ home TDD by 20%[b]
Hypoglycemia within the past 24 h: Glucose 50–70 mg/dL (2.8–3.9 mmol/L)	↓ home TDD by 30%[b]
Hypoglycemia within the past 24 h: Glucose <50 mg/dL (2.8 mmol/L)	↓ home TDD by 40%[b]

TDD, total daily dose
[a]These recommendations are based on the algorithm developed by the Duke University Medical Center Glycemic Safety Committee
[b]Always consider making further adjustments if the patient continues to develop hypoglycemia despite changes

Scenario 3: Patient with Type 2 Diabetes Who Is Not Using Insulin and Is Not Hyperglycemic in the Hospital

This situation can occur in patients with type 2 diabetes who are overnourished at home but who are admitted after periods of fasting, as in gastrointestinal illnesses, or who have had moderate weight loss related to illness or other factors. Patients who are not hyperglycemic can be followed with glucose monitoring alone, at least four times daily, usually before meals and at bedtime. However, a scheduled insulin regimen must be added if glucoses rise above the target ranges. It is not appropriate to follow hyperglycemia with only a correctional insulin scale; this retroactive approach does not effectively prevent future hyperglycemic episodes and will increase the risk for hypoglycemia.

Insulin for Patients with Renal Impairment

For patients with renal impairment, it often is necessary to decrease the TDD depending on the stage of kidney failure due in large part to changes in insulin clearance (Table 2.2). This applies to patients with both chronic and acute renal failure, although patients with improving renal function after acute failure may have increasing insulin requirements. As always, prompt adjustments should be made according to monitored glucoses.

Table 2.2 Renal impairment warranting cautious modification of total daily dose[a]

Situation	Modification
Patient on insulin at home, no history of hypoglycemia, and stable CKD stage I and II (GFR >40 mL/min per BSA 1.73 m^2)	None: May use home TDD
CKD stage III (GFR 30–39 mL/min per BSA 1.73 m^2)	↓ home TDD by 30%
CKD stage IV (GFR 15–29 mL/min per BSA 1.73 m^2)	↓home TDD by 50%
CKD stage V (GFR 15 mL/min per BSA 1.73 m^2) or ESRD or acute renal injury	↓home TDD by 60%

BSA, body surface area; CKD, chronic kidney disease; ESRD, end-stage renal disease; GFR, glomerular filtration rate; TDD, total daily dose
[a]These recommendations are based on the algorithm developed by the Duke University Medical Center Glycemic Safety Committee

Insulin for Patients Taking Glucocorticoids

For patients taking glucocorticoids, it is recommended by some diabetologists that regular (Novolin R®, Humulin R®) insulin be used in order to adjust for the delayed increase in prandial glucose that may be seen in this scenario. In patients taking glucocorticoids, the fasting glucose may be minimally increased, with a substantially more exaggerated increase in postprandial glucose. Occasionally, patients without a previous diagnosis of diabetes might require only prandial insulin. As with other patients with hyperglycemia, the insulin dose should be based on the patient's weight, calorie consumption, meal time, and other associated factors that might be affecting glycemic levels (e.g., the patient's status following major surgical intervention).

Distribution of the Total Daily Dose

Most experts agree that a basal-bolus insulin regimen is the best approach for patients requiring intensive insulin treatment. The variable timing of nutrition, medications, and procedures in the hospital makes premixed and split-mix insulin regimens unreliable and dangerous. Basal-bolus insulin regimens will be different for patients who are eating regular, discrete meals than for those who have continuous nutrition (through EN or TPN routes) and those who are fasting.

The Patient Who Is Eating Discrete Meals

A basal-bolus regimen for this patient can be accomplished in two ways: (1) a long-acting peakless insulin (i.e., glargine [Lantus®] or detemir [Levemir®]), for the basal component with a rapid-acting insulin (i.e., aspart [Novolog®], lispro [Humalog®], or glulisine [apidra®]) at mealtime, or (2) an intermediate-acting insulin (i.e., NPH [Neutral Protamine Hagedorn]) at bedtime with a short-acting insulin (i.e., regular [Novolin R® or Humulin R]) at mealtime.

Long-Acting Insulin (Glargine[Lantus] or Detemir[Levemir]), with Rapid-Acting Insulin (Aspart[Novolog], Lispro[Humalog], or Glulisine[Apidra])

Long-acting insulin serves as the entire basal component; 50% of the TDD usually is administered as one or two long-acting insulin injections over 24 h. (If this component is greater than 50 units, it is advisable to give it as two injections to maximize absorption). This can be done at the same time or divided into morning and evening doses, according to the physician and patient preferences. The remaining 50% of the dose is divided into three mealtime injections of rapid-acting insulin such that approximately 17% is administered at each meal. It should be noted that this equal distribution of mealtime doses must be adjusted subsequently based on glucose levels; it is rare for a patient to consume equal amounts of carbohydrates for each meal of the day. If the patient skips a meal, rapid-acting insulin should not be given.

Although a basal insulin such as glargine or detemir can be given at any time of the day, it is commonly given at bedtime, in part to prevent the mistake of mixing it with a short- or rapid-acting insulin.

Intermediate-Acting Insulin (NPH[Neutral Protamine Hagedorn]), and Short-Acting Insulin (Regular [Novolin R or Humulin R])

In this strategy, the basal and bolus components are not distinctly divided into separate insulins. Thus, the role of each insulin is not as intuitive as with the long- and rapid-acting insulins. Nonetheless, the strategy is simple. Here, 25% of the TDD is administered as short-acting (regular) insulin before each of the three meals. The remaining 25% is administered as intermediate-acting (NPH) insulin at bedtime.

An important feature of this type of plan is that, unlike the long- and rapid-acting insulin plan, mealtime insulin must be given even when a meal is omitted or reduced. This is because the mealtime insulin covers part of the basal-insulin requirement. When a patient is fasting, the "mealtime" insulin dose should be reduced by half, and the full bedtime dose should be continued unchanged (see below). Additionally, it is important to consider proper timing of the short-acting insulin in relation to meals. The most challenging aspect of this regimen in the inpatient setting is to ensure the delivery of short-acting insulin 30–45 min before a meal, for optimal efficacy.

NPH insulin has a significant peak, albeit fairly broad, which means it has a bolus component as well. Therefore, in some people, it may be helpful when given in the morning, to help cover lunch, and given at bedtime to help with the dawn hepatic glucose output surge. However, for patients who are fasting and who do not exhibit this dawn phenomenon, the dose of evening NPH must be reduced to prevent hypoglycemia. Furthermore, NPH insulin is not recommended for daytime use for patients who are fasting, as the midday peak may result in hypoglycemia.

The Patient Who Is Not Eating

The general principal in this situation is to continue the basal component while removing the bolus component. For the long- and rapid-acting insulin strategy described above, the long-acting insulin can be continued at the usual dose and time. The rapid-acting insulin is not given. When used at an appropriate dose, basal insulin should not cause fasting hypo- or hyperglycemia. However, for patients who will have prolonged periods of fasting or whose basal dose is unknown, administration of a long-acting basal insulin may increase the risk for prolonged hypoglycemia, and use is not recommended. These patients can be transitioned to a regimen of regular insulin every 6 h, as below. For the intermediate- and short-acting insulin regimen, the regimen can be changed in two ways. If the period of fasting is short-term, the existing regimen can be continued, with administration of half doses of the regular insulin at mealtimes. Alternatively, for patients who are not eating for an extended period of time, short-acting (regular) insulin may be given every 6 h without any intermediate-acting (NPH) insulin. In this second strategy, there will still be a small peak in the insulin activity, but it prevents hyperglycemia similar to longer-acting basal insulin, without the danger of prolonged hypoglycemia.

Patients with type 1 diabetes should always receive basal insulin, even if they are not eating, to prevent development of DKA. If necessary, IV dextrose (D5) may be given to support blood glucose during this time.

Correctional Insulin Scale

The correctional insulin scale is a tool designed to correct unpredictable hyperglycemia so that a patient's scheduled insulin regimen can be effective. It should not be used alone. Importantly, correctional insulin is given as a rapid- or short-acting insulin along with bolus insulin (depending on the patient's scheduled insulin type); it should never be given at bedtime.

Although many institutions have a "standard" correctional insulin scale, it is better to calculate an individualized scale to avoid under- or overtreatment. A quick and easy estimation for the scale increment is to use 5% of the TDD of insulin. For

Table 2.3 Example of correctional insulin scale

Glucose	Correctional insulin dose[a]
150 mg/dL (8.0 mmol/L)	None
150–200 mg/dL (8.0–11.0 mmol/L)	3 units
201–250 mg/dL (11.1–13.8 mmol/L)	6 units
251–300 mg/dL (13.9–16.6 mmol/L)	9 units
>300 mg/dL (>16.6 mmol/L)	12 units

[a]In some patients it might be too aggressive to start a correctional insulin scale at 150 mg/dL (8.0 mmol/L); e.g. a patient with hypoglycemia unawareness

example, if a patient has a TDD of 60, then 5% of 60 units is 3 units. Thus, the scale is designed with 3-unit increments as shown in Table 2.3.

Key Points: Choosing an Insulin Regimen

- All of the calculations shown here are estimates. Each patient will have a unique response to insulin, which will vary with inpatient circumstances. Thus, it is critical to reassess the regimen daily and adjust promptly. If this becomes challenging, an endocrine consultant can assist.
- Calculate a weight-based TDD of insulin for a starting point, or use the home TDD, if it appears reasonable.
- Make modifications based on age, type of diabetes, concern for hypoglycemia, use of non-insulin antidiabetic agents, renal function, and concomitant glucocorticoid use.
- Divide into basal and bolus components and, if desired, add a correctional insulin scale.

Bibliography

American Diabetes Association. Diabetes care executive summary from the American Diabetes Association. Standards of medical care in diabetes 2009. *Diabetes Care.* 2009;32(suppl 1): S6–S12.

Campbell KB, Braithwaite S. Hospital management of hyperglycemia. *Clin Diabetes.* 2004;22(2):81–88.

Clement S, Braithwaite SS, Magee MF, et al. Management of diabetes and hyperglycemia in hospitals. *Diabetes Care.* 2004; 27(2):553–591.

Hamann A, Matthaei S, Rosak C, Silvestre L for the HOE901/4007 Study Group. A randomized clinical trial comparing breakfast, dinner, or bedtime administration of insulin glargine in patients with type 1 diabetes. *Diabetes Care.* 2003; 26(6):1738–1744.

Hirsch I, Pauw D, Brunzell J. Inpatient management of adults with diabetes. *Diabetes Care.* 1995; 18(6):870–878.

Inzucchi SE. Management of hyperglycemia in the hospital setting. *N Engl J Med.* 2006; 355(18):1903–1911.

Kitabchi A, Freirea A, Umpierrez G. Evidence for strict inpatient blood glucose control: time to revise glycemic goals in hospitalized patients. *Metabolism.* 2008; 57(1):116–120.

Levetan C, Magee M. Hospital management of diabetes. *Endocrinol Metab Clin N Am.* 2000; 29(4):745–770.

Lien LF, Bethel MA, Feinglos MN. In-hospital management of type 2 diabetes mellitus. *Med Clin N Am.* 2004;88(4):1085–1105, xii.

Moghissi ES, Korytkowski MT, DiNardo M. American Association of Clinical Endocrinologist and American Diabetes Association consensus statement on inpatient glycemic control. *Endocr Pract.* 2009;15(4):1–17.

Nathan D. Insulin treatment of type 2 diabetes mellitus. In: Prote D, Sherwin R, Baron A, eds. *Ellenberg and Rifkin's Diabetes Mellitus.* 6th ed. New York, NY: McGraw-Hill; 2003:515–522.

NICE-SUGAR Study Investigators. Intensive versus conventional glucose control in critically ill patients. *N Engl J Med.* 2009;360(13):1283–1297.

Trence DL. Management of patients on chronic glucocorticoid therapy: an endocrine perspective. *Prim Care.* 2003;30(3):593–605.

Umpierrez GE, Andres P, Smiley D, et al. Randomized study of basal-bolus insulin therapy in the inpatient management of patients with type 2 diabetes (Rabbit 2 trial). *Diabetes Care.* 2007;30(9):2181–2186.

Umpierrez GE, Palacio A, Smiley D. Sliding scale insulin dose: myth or insanity. *Am J Med.* 2007;120(7):563–567 (Review).

Wesorick D, O'Malley C, Rushakoff R, Larsen K, Magee M. Management of diabetes and hyperglycemia in the hospital: a practical guide to subcutaneous insulin use in the non-critically ill, adult patient. *J Hosp Med.* 2008;3(suppl 5):S17–S28.

Wittlin S, Woehrle H, Gerich J. Insulin pharmacokinetics. In: Leahy J, Cefalu W, eds. *Insulin Therapy.* New York, NY: Marcel Dekker; 2002:73–85.

Chapter 3
IV Insulin Infusions: How to Use an "Insulin Drip"

Melanie E. Mabrey and Lillian F. Lien

Keywords IV insulin · Diabetic ketoacidosis · Hyperosmolar nonketotic hyperglycemia

Appropriate Scenarios for Use

Several clinical scenarios mandate the use of an IV insulin infusion (often informally referred to as an "insulin drip"). Any inpatient with diabetic ketoacidosis (DKA) requires an IV insulin infusion for proper management; simply continuing subcutaneous injections is not the standard of care in the hospital. Also, a patient with hyperosmolar nonketotic hyperglycemia should be initially managed with IV insulin. Indeed, any critically ill patient with persistent hyperglycemia for 24 h is a candidate for an IV insulin infusion, particularly if the hyperglycemia lingers despite increasing doses of subcutaneous insulin. Many surgical units now consider IV insulin to be the standard of care in patients with diabetes during the perioperative period, based on the data that glycemic control decreases the risk for infection and improves morbidity and mortality in the surgical patient. Common indications for uses of IV insulin can be found in Table 3.1.

NOTE: A single dose of IV insulin as a bolus is only appropriate in two settings: when starting an insulin infusion and for temporary treatment of hyperkalemia. It is almost *never* sufficient to give a bolus of IV insulin without simultaneously starting an IV insulin infusion. The half-life of IV insulin is only minutes; once given, the insulin will be cleared within 20 minutes in patients with normal renal function. This rapid clearance is the reason that an IV bolus alone is not effective.

Key Points: Scenarios for Use

- Use IV insulin for a patient with DKA or hyperosmolar nonketotic hyperglycemia, and consider it for any acutely ill patient (Table 3.1).

M.E. Mabrey (✉)
Duke Inpatient Diabetes Management, Department of Advanced Clinical Practice, Duke University Hospital, Durham, NC, USA; Duke University Schools of Nursing and Medicine, Duke University Medical Center, Durham, NC, USA
e-mail: mabre002@mc.duke.edu

L.F. Lien et al. (eds.), *Glycemic Control in the Hospitalized Patient*,
DOI 10.1007/978-1-60761-006-9_3, © Springer Science+Business Media, LLC 2011

- Apart from emergent hyperkalemia treatment, never use a single IV insulin bolus without simultaneously starting an IV insulin infusion.
- IV insulin has a very short half-life.

Table 3.1 Common indications for the uses of IV insulin

- Diabetic ketoacidosis
- Hyperosmolar nonketotic hyperglycemia
- Persistent hyperglycemia, uncontrolled by subcutaneous insulin
- Myocardial infarction
- Dose finding in patients with glycemic lability
- Hyperglycemia in high-dose corticosteroids
- Labor and delivery
- Peri- and postoperative glycemic management
- Temporary, severe hyperglycemia induced by acute illness
- Temporary, severe hyperglycemia induced by medications (i.e., glucocorticoids)

Starting the IV Insulin Infusion

IV insulin infusions are dosed in units per hour, based on weight in kilograms (see Table 3.2). Regular insulin is the type most commonly prescribed for IV use. Although there are anecdotal reports of rapid-acting types of insulin given via this route, the efficacy and safety of these newer insulins in this setting are not well studied.

Table 3.2 Initial IV insulin infusion rate calculations

Patient	Initial infusion rate	Bolus dose
DKA	0.1 units/kg/h	0.1 units/kg given as a single bolus prior to starting the IV infusion (ADULTS only)
Any setting other than DKA	0.025 units/kg/h	May provide a 0.025 units/kg single bolus when starting the IV insulin

Bedside glucose monitoring should be performed hourly for the patient on IV insulin until stable. Once blood glucoses have been stable for four consecutive hours, some providers may allow some leniency in monitoring (i.e., glucose checks every 2 h) but the default should always be hourly monitoring in an unstable patient.

Insulin is a major regulator of potassium via the sodium-potassium pump. Prior to initiating IV insulin, the patient's potassium level must be assessed. IV insulin should not be started without treatment of the potassium if the level is less than 3.3 mEq/L. On the other hand, for hyperkalemic patients, IV insulin will assist with transport of potassium into the cell. For details on the management of electrolytes in DKA, see Chapter 6: Hyperglycemic Emergencies.

Adjusting the IV Insulin Infusion Rates

A number of protocols have been developed to assist with titration of IV insulin infusion rates, and most hospitals have a preferred order set. We favor an insulin infusion nomogram that takes into account the patient's insulin-sensitivity level. One way to achieve this is to adjust the insulin infusion according to the rate of change of glucose level from hour to hour. A multiplication factor can be used to assist with titration: An example of this type of protocol is the Lien-Spratt IV insulin nomogram used throughout Duke University Hospital (Fig. 3.1). Implementation of this nomogram was found to significantly reduce errors in the delivery of IV insulin, which also reduced episodes of persistent hyperglycemia in critical care patients.

Other IV insulin protocols account for differences in patients' insulin sensitivities by using a choice format (with the appropriate algorithm chosen according to level of sensitivity). In any case, a safe general goal for treatment of hyperglycemia with IV insulin is an hourly decrease in blood glucose of approximately 50–75 mg/dL (2.7–4.1 mmol/L). Overall, the choice of protocol is less important than ensuring that a single method of titrating IV insulin is used throughout the institution and that providers and staff are all educated on how to properly adhere to the protocol to promote safety. If there is uncertainty about the method at the institution, the charge nurse on the patient's nursing unit should be consulted.

Despite the effectiveness of IV insulin protocols for most patients, it is worth noting that there are patients for whom no protocol is perfect. An example is the highly insulin-resistant patient, who may require large volumes of IV insulin (e.g., >20 units/h). Similarly, the highly insulin-sensitive patient, particularly those with renal failure and type 1 diabetes, may require very small volumes of insulin. This type of patient will require the attention of an experienced provider (rather than a protocol alone), and when an endocrinology consultation is available, it should be requested.

Key Points: Implementation of IV Insulin

- Start the infusion at a weight-based dose rate (Table 3.2).
- Titrate the dose according to the institution's protocol (Fig. 3.1), including frequent glucose monitoring.

Special Scenario: IV Insulin in the Patient Who Is Eating

If the patient is ready to start eating regular food but still requires an insulin infusion, the IV insulin infusion will cover basal insulin needs, but will generally not be effective for the patient's prandial hyperglycemia. Thus, a reasonable strategy is to

DUKE UNIVERSITY HOSPITAL
INSULIN INTRAVENOUS NOMOGRAM
AND ORDER SET (LIEN-SPRATT METHOD)

M05JB (9/04)

© 2004 Duke University Medical Center
All rights reserved.
Used with permission.

STEP 1. Starting the Insulin Drip:
- ☐ If patient is not in DKA: Weight of patient in kilograms (kg) _____ X 0.025 units = _____ units/hour
- ☐ If patient is in DKA: Weight of patient in kilograms (kg) _____ X 0.1 units = _____ units/hour
- ☐ If patient's glucose < 160 (i.e. acute MI protocol), then start drip at 1 unit/hour

STEP 2. Check blood glucose (BG) hourly and record. Adjust insulin infusion rate per table below.
- ☒ Notify MD, if any BG is less than 85 mg/dl or greater than 450 mg/dl

STEP 3. Medications and Fluids   Also see BACK page for more info
- ☐ 1000ml D5W with _____ mEq KCl at _____ mL/hour.   ☒ Infuse insulin and IV fluids on separate pumps
- ☐ Other IV/DKA fluids: _____   infuse at _____ mL/hour
- ☒ Pharmacy to prepare human regular insulin 250 units in 250 ml NS (1 unit/ml)
- ☒ Titrate insulin infusion as follows:

STEP 4. NURSE: MULTIPLY CURRENT INSULIN RATE BY NUMBER BELOW. RESULT IS NEW INSULIN RATE IN UNITS/HOUR.

If Current BG =	If Prior BG =	Multiply current insulin rate by # below
Any BG < 85	Stop insulin and notify MD	
85-100	< 120	0.6
	120-150	0.5
	151-200	0.3
	> 200	0.1
101-120	<100	1
	100-120	0.9
	121-140	0.7
	141-180	0.6
	181-225	0.5
	226-250	0.4
	251-275	0.3
	276-450	0.1
121-140	< 100	1.1
	100-140	1
	141-160	0.9
	161-180	0.8
	181-200	0.7
	201-225	0.5
	226-275	0.4
	276-300	0.3
	301-325	0.2
	326-450	0.1
141-160	<100	1.2
	100-140	1.1
	141-160	1
	161-180	0.9
	181-200	0.7
	201-225	0.6
	226-275	0.5
	276-300	0.4
	301-325	0.2
	326-450	0.1

If Current BG =	If Prior BG =	Multiply current insulin rate by # below
161-175	<100	1.4
	100-140	1.2
	141-175	1.1
	176-200	1
	201-225	0.9
	226-250	0.7
	251-275	0.5
	276-300	0.4
	301-350	0.2
	351-450	0.1
176-200	< 100	1.5
	100-200	1.2
	201-250	1
	251-275	0.7
	276-300	0.5
	301-325	0.4
	326-350	0.3
	351-450	0.2
201-225	< 100	1.5
	100-150	1.4
	151-200	1.3
	201-250	1.2
	251-275	1
	276-300	0.8
	301-325	0.5
	326-350	0.3
	351-450	0.2
226-250	< 100	1.8
	100-150	1.6
	151-225	1.4
	226-275	1.2
	276-300	1
	301-325	0.8
	326-350	0.5
	351-400	0.4
	401-450	0.2

If Current BG =	If Prior BG =	Multiply current insulin rate by # below
251-275	< 100	2
	100-150	1.8
	151-200	1.6
	201-275	1.4
	276-300	1.2
	301-325	1
	326-350	0.8
	351-400	0.5
	401-450	0.4
276-300	< 100	2.2
	100-200	1.8
	201-250	1.6
	251-300	1.4
	301-325	1.2
	326-375	1
	376-400	0.5
	401-450	0.4
301-325	< 100	2.4
	100-175	2
	176-250	1.8
	251-300	1.6
	301-325	1.4
	326-350	1.2
	351-400	1
	401-450	0.5

If Current BG =	If Prior BG =	Multiply current insulin rate by # below
326-350	< 100	2.6
	100-250	2
	251-275	1.8
	276-325	1.6
	326-350	1.4
	351-375	1.2
	376-450	1
351-375	< 100	2.8
	100-200	2.2
	201-275	2
	276-325	1.8
	326-350	1.6
	351-375	1.4
	376-450	1.2
376-400	< 100	3
	100-250	2.2
	251-325	2
	326-350	1.8
	351-375	1.6
	376-450	1.4
401-450	< 100	3.2
	100-200	2.4
	201-275	2.2
	276-350	2
	351-375	1.8
	376-450	1.6
> 450	Notify MD	

STEP 5. Monitoring
- ☒ Monitor bedside BG every 1 hour. Record hourly BG on the MAR and insulin drip rates on flowsheet
- ☒ When IV insulin is stopped, continue every 1 hour BG checks x 3 or until stable
- ☒ Begin hypoglycemic protocol for BG < 70 mg/dL and Notify HO
- ☒ Begin subcutaneous insulin one hour before stopping IV insulin when transitioning from IV to SC therapy

STEP 6. Consults and patient education ☐ Nutrition ☐ Diabetes Mgmt service 9▆▆▆ ☐ Diabetes CNS 9▆▆▆
STEP 7. Provider signature/Title/ID_____ : Date/time_____

White - Chart   Yellow - Pharmacy   Pink - Nursing

Fig. 3.1 (continued)

continue the IV infusion of regular insulin as before, titrated per the usual protocol, while also adding low-dose rapid-acting insulin given subcutaneously at each meal. Orders for this patient may appear as follows:

- Infuse IV regular (Novolin R® or Humulin R®) insulin. Titrate according to nomogram, using data from hourly blood glucose monitoring.

QUESTION	ANSWER
When should IV insulin be initiated? © 2004 **Duke University Medical Center** **All rights reserved.** **Used with permission.**	• In critically ill patient when BG > 250 x 24 hrs despite q 6 hr SQ insulin administration. • In critically ill patient when BG > 200 x 48 hrs despite active increase of q 6 hr SQ insulin administration. • In DKA when AG > 10 or serum acetone is positive.
How do I start the drip?	• **Start 0.025 units per kg/hour** for patients NOT in DKA (Also see DKA instructions below.)
What is the prior blood glucose (BG)?	The prior blood glucose is the blood glucose **in the hour prior** to the current blood glucose.
How **fast** should blood glucose drop?	Goal is for BG to drop approximately • 75 mg/dl an hour when BG > 275 and • 50 mg/dl an hour when BG < 275
What if the new insulin drip rate is not an integer?	• Round units to the nearest 1/10th of a unit; (e.g. 1.76 units becomes 1.8 units; 1.54 units becomes 1.5 units)
What should I do when there is a large **increase** in BG level (i.e. BG was 175, now 275)?	• Check infusion site • Check insulin drip for standard concentration • Assess for infection or new medication.
What should I do when **tube feeds** are held?	Decrease insulin dose by 75%, but the insulin drip should **not** be held.
Hypoglycemia (< 70 mg/dl)	• Hold infusion and notify physician • Begin hypoglycemia protocol; continue BG monitoring q1h • After infusion has been on hold, when BG > 100, discuss with physician about appropriate insulin infusion rate to restart. Physician should consider last 6 hours of insulin infusion rate data to determine the best restart rate.
When do I **discontinue** the drip?	When patient has a stable BG of < 150 for 4 to 6 hours and no new problems (i.e. fever, sepsis, new pressors, new tube feeds). Needs MD order.
How to **discontinue** the drip and **CONVERT** to SQ Insulin?	• Add up the total insulin units given over the past 24 hours. This is the **new total daily dose.** (You may want to consider decreasing slightly by 20%) • Give **1/4th** of the total daily dose as regular insulin SQ every 6 hours if NPO or on Tube Feeds. • If eating: Give **1/4th** of the total daily dose as regular insulin before meals and NPH insulin at bedtime • Remember, the first dose of SQ insulin should be given 1 hour before stopping IV insulin
Give SQ insulin 1 hour before drip is stopped	• Do **NOT STOP** IV Insulin without giving SQ Insulin.
When converting to SQ insulin, How do I calculate the **Supplemental Scale?** • Note this is different from a sliding scale where insulin is given only when BG is > 200 • You may want to request parameters for holding or Halving insulin if BG < 70 or BG < 100	Sliding Scale goes up by increments of 5% of total daily dose: Example: If patient is on a total of 100 units of insulin daily, then each increment is 5 units, so...the scale reads: Blood Glucose Supplemental Scale using Regular Insulin 70- 200 ADD NOTHING to scheduled insulin 201-250 ADD 5 units to normally scheduled insulin 251-300 ADD 10 units to normally scheduled insulin 301-350 ADD 15 units to normally scheduled insulin 351-400 ADD 20 units and notify MD
DKA Instructions	• Fluid expansion with **normal saline with KCL** as ordered by MD (K+ will be falsely high. Need MD order for KCL.) • Start drip at **0.1 units/kg/hour.** • Add D5 to NS when BG < 250mg/dl. • Continue insulin drip until anion gap and urine ketones have cleared.

Fig. 3.1 Duke University Hospital: Lien-Spratt IV insulin nomogram. Source: Lien et al. (2005). Reproduced with permission from Endocrine Practice and the American Association of Clinical Endocrinologists

- Give 6 units[1] of lispro (Humalog®) or aspart (Novolog®), or glulisine (Apidra®) insulin subcutaneously three times/day before meals only. Hold if patient is NPO (nothing by mouth).

Transitioning to Subcutaneous Insulin

The first important step is determining when it is safe to transition the patient from an IV to a subcutaneous insulin regimen. The patient may be ready for the transition if the following are in place:

- Stable blood glucoses between 140 and 180 mg/dL (7.7–10 mmol/L) for at least 4–6 h consecutively
- Normal anion gap
- Resolution of acidosis
- Stable clinical status
- Not on vasopressors
- Stable nutrition plan or patient is eating

Once a patient stabilizes insulin requirements may change dramatically, and it is prudent to monitor the glucose levels frequently, particularly when transitioning from IV to subcutaneous insulin.

Transitioning from IV to Subcutaneous Insulin in the NPO Patient

In the NPO patient, the conversion is fairly straightforward; it is reasonable to assume that the IV insulin infusion has accounted for the patient's basal needs.

Step 1: Calculate the 24-h IV insulin requirement. In other words, how much IV insulin does the patient need to maintain control over 24 h? Keep in mind that it may be necessary to estimate an average infusion rate based on a shorter period of time (such as between midnight and 6 AM) if the glucoses were the most stable during that period (Table 3.3).

Table 3.3 Insulin infusion rate example

Time	2100	2200	2300	MN	0100	0200	0300	0400	0500	0600
Glucose (mg/dL)	300	200	110	130	140	126	130	128	135	140
Insulin rate (units/h)	4.0	2.0	1.0	1.0	1.0	1.0	1.0	1.0	1.0	1.0

---

[1] The dose estimate for the subcutaneous rapid-acting insulin with meals should be fairly conservative, as many patients may be just beginning to resume food intake in this scenario. In general, we would recommend a dose of no more than 0.1 units/kg/day subcutaneously with each meal.

- Since the patient has had stable glucoses from midnight to 6 AM, this is a good time period to use for the calculation.
- During this time, the IV insulin infusion rate was 1 unit/h.
- Extrapolated to a 24-h period, 24 h × 1 unit/h = 24 units.
- *Thus, the 24-h IV insulin requirement is 24 units.*

Step 2: Calculate a total daily dose (TDD) of subcutaneous insulin. Typically, this will be a fraction of the 24-h IV insulin requirement. A safe estimate is 80% of the 24-h IV insulin requirement as the new TDD for subcutaneous insulin.

Example Continued

- Calculate 80% of 24 units = 19.2. For simplicity, round to 20 units.
- *Therefore, the TDD of subcutaneous insulin will be 20 units.*

Step 3: Decide how to distribute the subcutaneous insulin throughout the day. Because the patient is still NPO, a simple and safe regimen will be once-daily basal insulin (glargine [Lantus®] or detemir [Levemir®]) particularly in patients with a known history of diabetes.

Example Continued

The TDD of subcutaneous insulin is estimated at 20 units.

- For the patient with a known history of diabetes, a simple and safe regimen will be once-daily basal insulin. Thus, the patient would receive *20 units of basal insulin (glargine [Lantus®] or detemir [Levemir®]) given subcutaneously once daily.*
- For the patient without a history of diabetes, or when the provider is concerned about a potential reduction in insulin requirements over the next 24 h, the TDD is best divided into four injections of short-acting insulin:

  - 20 units/4 = 5 units per injection.
  - *Thus, the 4-injection subcutaneous regimen should be 5 units regular (Novolin R® or Humulin R®) insulin subcutaneously every 6 h.*

Transitioning from IV to Subcutaneous Insulin in the Patient Already Eating

Option 1: Transition to Long-acting Basal and Rapid-acting Prandial Insulin

The goal in this situation is to create a basal–bolus (4-injection) subcutaneous insulin regimen, mimicking physiologic insulin production, using

- Rapid-acting insulin lispro (Humalog®) or aspart (Novolog®), or glulisine (apidra®) subcutaneously three times a day with meals, and

- Long-acting insulin (glargine [Lantus®] or detemir [Levemir®]) subcutaneously at bedtime.

Because the patient is already eating, he or she should already be on a combination of IV insulin for basal needs and rapid-acting subcutaneous insulin at each meal for prandial needs, as in the section above on administration of IV insulin to the patient who is eating.

Step 1: Prandial Insulin

- If the rapid-acting subcutaneous insulin already begun was adjusted appropriately, then this can simply be continued three times a day with meals.
- Example: If the patient already is receiving 6 units of rapid-acting subcutaneous insulin three times a day before meals, this regimen should be continued.

Step 2: Basal Insulin

- Calculate the 24-h IV insulin requirement in the same manner as described in the NPO section.
- Again, use only 80% of this 24-h IV insulin requirement as the subcutaneous basal dose.

EXAMPLE

- Patient with a 24-h IV insulin requirement of 24 units.
- Calculate 80% of 24 units = 19.2. For simplicity, round to 20 units.
- Therefore, the basal dose of subcutaneous insulin will be 20 units.

Step 3: The above steps should complete the basal–bolus regimen.

- EXAMPLE: Final orders should read as follows:
- *6 units of rapid-acting insulin subcutaneously three times a day with meals*
- *20 units of long-acting insulin subcutaneously at bedtime.*

A word of caution: The above simple transition is appropriate if the IV insulin is truly only covering basal needs. If there is any concern that the IV insulin may also be covering prandial needs, then the first step is to titrate up the prandial subcutaneous insulin accordingly, and lower the IV requirement, *before* attempting a transition.

Transitioning from IV to Subcutaneous Insulin in the Patient Already Eating

Option 2: Transition to Regular and NPH Subcutaneous Insulin

The goal in this situation is to create an intensive basal–bolus (4-injection) subcutaneous insulin regimen using the following:

- Regular insulin subcutaneously three times a day before meals, and
- NPH insulin subcutaneously at bedtime.

Because the patient is already eating, he or she should be on a combination of IV insulin for basal needs and rapid-acting subcutaneous insulin at each meal for prandial needs, as in the section above on IV Insulin in the patient who is eating.

Step 1: Prandial Insulin

- If the rapid-acting subcutaneous insulin already begun was adjusted appropriately, this can simply be added up to determine the total prandial dose.
- EXAMPLE: The patient already receiving 6 units of rapid-acting subcutaneous insulin three times a day before meals is receiving a total of 18 units of prandial insulin.

Step 2: Basal Insulin

- Calculate the 24-h IV insulin requirement in the same manner as described in the NPO section.
- Again, use only 80% of this 24-h IV insulin requirement as the subcutaneous basal dose.

EXAMPLE

- Patient with a 24-h IV insulin requirement of 24 units.
- Calculate 80% of 24 units = 19.2. For simplicity, round to 20 units.
- Therefore, the basal dose of subcutaneous insulin will be 20 units.

Step 3: Total the TDD of insulin

- EXAMPLE: From above, if the patient has a prandial subcutaneous insulin requirement of 18 units plus a basal subcutaneous insulin requirement of 20 units, he or she will need *38 units as the TDD for subcutaneous insulin.*

Step 4: Redistribute the TDD as regular and NPH subcutaneous insulin

- 25% of the TDD (1/4 TDD) is administered as regular insulin before breakfast, before lunch, and before dinner.

- 25% of the TDD (1/4 TDD) is administered as NPH insulin before bedtime.

EXAMPLE: The above calculation showed a TDD of 38 units of subcutaneous insulin. Therefore, 1/4 TDD = 9.5 rounded to 10 units.

- Final orders should read as below:

    - *10 units regular insulin subcutaneously three times daily with meals.*
    - *10 units NPH insulin subcutaneously at bedtime.*

Overlap of IV Insulin Discontinuation and Subcutaneous Insulin Initiation

The first subcutaneous insulin dose should be administered at least 1 h *before* stopping the IV insulin infusion. This is particularly critical for patients with impaired insulin secretion as in type 1 diabetes or long-standing type 2 diabetes. This is important because all subcutaneous insulin has a time to onset that is longer than the half-life of the IV insulin (<10 min). Failure to allow for overlap in the IV and subcutaneous insulin can result in rapid development of hyperglycemia. Thus, the subcutaneous insulin should be given as follows:

- 1 h before discontinuation of IV insulin when using regular or rapid-acting subcutaneous insulin.
- 3–6 h before discontinuing IV insulin when using intermediate or long-acting subcutaneous insulin.

Bibliography

Bode BW, Braithwaite SS, Steed DR, Davidson PC. Intravenous insulin infusion therapy: indications, methods, and transition to subcutaneous insulin therapy. *Endocr Pract.* 2004;10(suppl 2):71–80.

Brown G, Dodek P. Intravenous insulin nomogram improves blood glucose control in the critically ill. *Crit Care Med.* 2001;29(9):1714–1719.

Clement S, Braithwaite S, Magee M, et al. Management of diabetes and hyperglycemia in hospitals. *Diabetes Care.* 2004;27(2):553–591.

Davis ED, Harwood K, Midgett L, Mabrey M, Lien LF. Implementation of a new intravenous insulin method on intermediate-care units in hospitalized patients. *Diabetes Educ.* 2005;31(6): 818–821, 823.

Furnary AP, Gao G, Grunkemeier GL, et al. Continuous insulin infusion reduces mortality in patients with diabetes undergoing coronary artery bypass grafting. *J Thorac Cardiovasc Surg.* 2003; 125(5):1007–1021.

Furnary AP, Zerr KJ, Grunkemeier GL, Starr A. Continuous insulin infusion reduces the incidence of deep sternal wound infection in diabetic patients after cardiac surgical procedures. *Ann Thorac Surg.* 1999;67(2):352–362.

Goldberg PA, Siegel MD, Sherwin RS, et al. Implementation of a safe and effective insulin infusion protocol in a medical intensive care unit. *Diabetes Care.* 2004;27(2):461–467.

Henderson KE, Baranski TJ, Bickel PE, Clutter WE, McGill JB, eds. *The Washington Manual Endocrinology Subspecialty Consult*. 2nd ed. Philadelphia, PA: Lippincott Williams & Wilkins; 2009.

Krinsley JS. Effect of an intensive glucose management protocol on the mortality of critically ill adult patients. *Mayo Clin Proc*. 2004;79(8):992–1000.

Lien L, Bethel MA, Feinglos M. In-hospital management of type 2 diabetes mellitus. *Med Clin North Am*. 2004;88(4):1085–1105.

Lien LF, Spratt SE, Woods Z, Osborne K, Feinglos MN. Optimizing hospital use of intravenous insulin: improved hyperglycemic management and error reduction with a new nomogram. *Endocr Pract*. 2005;11(4):240–253.

Malmberg K, Ryden L, Efendic S, et al. Randomized trial of insulin-glucose infusion followed by subcutaneous insulin treatment in diabetic patients with acute myocardial infarction (DIGAMI Study): effects on mortality at 1 year. *J Am Coll Cardiol*. 1995;26(1):57–65.

Markovitz LJ, Wiechmann RJ, Harris N, et al. Description and evaluation of a glycemic management protocol for patients with diabetes undergoing heart surgery. *Endocr Pract*. 2002;8(1):10–18.

Moghissi ES, Korytkowski MT, DiNardo M, et al. American Association of Clinical Endocrinologists and American Diabetes Association consensus statement on inpatient glycemic control. *Endocr Pract*. 2009;15(4):353–369.

Nazer LH, Chow SL, Moghissi ES. Insulin infusion protocols for critically ill patients: a highlight of differences and similarities. *Endocr Pract*, 2007;13(2):137–146.

Trence DL, Kelly JL, Hirsch IB. The rationale and management of hyperglycemia for inpatients with cardiovascular disease: time for change. *J Clin Endocrinol Metab*. 2003;88(6):2430–2437.

Umpierrez GE, Jones S, Smiley D, et al. Insulin analogs versus human insulin in the treatment of patients with diabetic ketoacidosis: a randomized controlled trial. *Diabetes Care*. 2009;32(7):1164–1169.

Van den Berghe G, Wouters P, Weekers F, et al. Intensive insulin therapy in the critically ill patient. *N Engl J Med*. 2001;345(19):1359–1367.

Zerr KJ, Furnary AP, Grunkemeier GL, Bookin S, Kanhere V, Starr A. Glucose control lowers the risk of wound infection in diabetics after open heart operation. *Ann Thorac Surg*. 1997;63(2):356–361.

Chapter 4
Laboratory Testing in Hospitalized Patients with Diabetes Mellitus

Karen Barnard and Mary E. Cox

Keywords Random plasma glucose · Fasting plasma glucose · Oral glucose tolerance test · Point-of-care glucose test (POCT) · Hemoglobin A_{1C} · Fructosamine · Insulin · Pro-insulin · C-peptide · Autoantibody · Ketone · Urine microalbumin · Lipid panel · High sensitivity CRP (hsCRP)

Many of the laboratory tests routinely ordered for patients with diabetes mellitus in the outpatient setting are of more limited use in the hospitalized patient. However, the hospital is certainly a place for opportunistic diabetes diagnosis, and laboratory monitoring for effects of therapy is essential. The laboratory tests that are most useful for management of an inpatient with diabetes are discussed in this chapter (Table 4.1).

Glucose-Based Tests

Plasma Glucose

Plasma glucose is obtained by venipuncture and is conveniently assayed with other components of the basic metabolic panel. In order to avoid falsely low readings, plasma glucose samples must be processed promptly. In the hospital, uses of plasma glucose include the following: (1) provision of support to a new diabetes diagnosis, (2) monitoring effectiveness of therapy in patients for whom point-of-care glucose testing (POCT) is unreliable, and (3) confirmation of an extreme POCT glucose value obtained from a portable glucose meter. The following sections review diabetes screening and diagnostic testing, as well as POCT.

K. Barnard (✉)
Division of Endocrinology, Metabolism, and Nutrition, Department of Medicine, Duke University Medical Center, Durham, NC 27710, USA; Department of Veterans Affairs, Durham, NC 27707, USA
e-mail: karen.barnard@duke.edu

Table 4.1 Laboratory tests for inpatient diabetes assessment

Test	Recommended for routine inpatient use	Inpatient use	Limitations to use
Plasma glucose	Yes	Opportunistic or intentional diabetes diagnosis; confirmation of extreme point-of-care glucose levels	Limited for diabetes diagnosis because of propensity toward circumstantial variability; sample requires prompt processing
Point-of-care glucose	Yes	Routine monitoring of glucose-lowering therapy	May be inaccurate at extreme glucose levels
Urinary glucose	No	Not recommended	Not recommended
A$_{1C}$	Yes	Evidence-based monitoring of glucose-lowering therapy; diabetes diagnosis	Hospitalized patients may have reasons for inaccuracy
Point-of-care A$_{1C}$	No	Not recommended	Similar inaccuracy as for central laboratory A$_{1C}$; may measure slightly higher A$_{1C}$ values and may have additional intra- and interindividual variability
Fructosamine	No	Estimate overall effects of glucose-lowering therapy for patients in whom A$_{1C}$ is unreliable	Little evidence correlating fructosamine level to complications and outcomes; highly variable
Markers of endogenous insulin (C-peptide, pro-insulin)	No	Hypoglycemia evaluation; limited use for diagnosis of type 1 diabetes	Can be unreliable in hyperglycemic emergencies and early type 1 diabetes
Insulin	No	Hypoglycemia evaluation	Not a reliable measure of endogenous insulin production and has high inter- and intraindividual variation
Autoantibody markers	No	Support of diagnosis of type 1 diabetes	Expensive and often unnecessary
Serum ketones	Yes, if DKA suspected	Support of diagnosis of DKA	May be falsely negative
Urine ketones	Yes, if DKA suspected	Support of diagnosis of DKA	May be positive in conditions other than DKA
Urine microalbumin	No	Diagnosis of diabetic nephropathy (>1 positive measurement)	Multiple causes of microalbuminuria other than diabetic nephropathy
Lipid panel	Yes	Cardiovascular risk stratification and monitoring of lipid-lowering therapy	May have falsely low levels in acute illness
hsCRP	No	Cardiovascular risk stratification	Unreliable in most hospitalized patients, particularly those with infectious and inflammatory conditions

DKA, diabetic ketoacidosis; hsCRP, high-sensitivity C-reactive protein

Diabetes Screening and Diagnosis

The screening and diagnostic criteria for diabetes are the same for inpatients as for outpatients, although all glucose-based tests share a fundamental flaw when used in the hospital: patient glucose levels can change considerably under the conditions of dietary alteration, physiologic stress, and disrupted sleep that often accompany hospital visits. Furthermore, there is no finite *physiologic* threshold for any diabetes diagnostic test at which normality ends and diabetes begins. All patients with risk factors for type 2 diabetes, even those with test parameters below the diagnostic thresholds, should be given appropriate education about nutrition, exercise, and weight loss. Results close to the diagnostic thresholds should be confirmed once the patient is stable and, preferably, an outpatient.

There are three categories of plasma glucose-based tests for screening and diagnosis of diabetes: (1) random plasma glucose (RPG), (2) fasting plasma glucose (FPG), and (3) oral glucose tolerance test (OGTT), discussed here in the context of a 75-g glucose load.

Random Plasma Glucose

The RPG is the most conveniently obtained, usually along with routine basic metabolic panels. The commonly held RPG threshold for diagnosis of diabetes is 200 mg/dL or greater (≥ 11.1 mmol/L), along with symptoms of polyuria, polydipsia, and unexplained weight loss. An RPG of 140–199 mg/dL (7.7–11 mmol/L) is suggestive of prediabetes. Based on diagnosis by OGTT, an RPG 200 mg/dL or greater (≥ 11.1 mmol/L) is insensitive but has a specificity approaching 100%, which, in the setting of symptoms, is unlikely to lead to a false-positive diagnosis. One must use caution, however, when diagnosing diabetes based on the RPG level given its propensity to change as a patient's circumstances do. Elevated levels should always be confirmed.

Fasting Plasma Glucose

The FPG test is a simple plasma glucose measurement obtained after at least 8 h of fasting (usually an overnight fast), which can be accomplished under supervision in the hospital. It has been the American Diabetes Association's (ADA) test of choice for diagnosis of both prediabetes (FPG 100–125 mg/dL [5.5–6.9 mmol/L]) and diabetes (FPG ≥ 126 [≥ 7 mmol/L]). Although the intraindividual stability is fair, FPG should be confirmed on a second occasion or with a second test to avoid false results.

Oral Glucose Tolerance Test

The 75-g OGTT currently is considered the worldwide gold standard for diabetes diagnosis. The 2-h post-load glucose level diagnostic for prediabetes is 140–199 mg/dL (7.7–11 mmol/L), and the level diagnostic for diabetes is $\geq$ at least

200 mg/dL ($\geq$11.1 mmol/L). OGTT is the only way to formally diagnose impaired glucose tolerance (IGT), which represents the fundamental pathophysiologic defect in type 2 diabetes (i.e., the inability to respond to insulin release). In the hospital, OGTT also has obvious practical downsides, such as the required 8-h fast before testing, commitment of nursing staff, and the length of the test itself.

POCT Glucose

POCT glucose, or capillary glucose, is measured by a portable glucose meter and measures whole blood glucose. POCT is used frequently in the hospital because of ease of use and rapidity of results. POCT glucose measurements are increasingly used to make point-of-care decisions about therapy. In general, use of these meters is reasonable; however, there are important limitations.

- POCT glucose is less reliable than plasma glucose when measuring extreme values, that is, less than 60 mg/dL (3.3 mmol/L) and greater than 500 mg/dL (27.7 mmol/L). Glucose levels in these ranges should be confirmed with plasma glucose.
- POCT glucose can differ by 10–15% from plasma glucose; the direction and magnitude of this difference varies among meters.
- Caution should be used in patients on peritoneal dialysis or in those receiving therapeutic immunoglobulin preparations. Many POCT testing kits employ the chemical glucose dehydrogenase pyrroloquinoline quinone (GDH-PQQ) to quantify glucose. GDH-PQQ reacts with several nonglucose sugars, including maltose, galactose, and xylose, which are found in peritoneal dialysis solutions and therapeutic immunoglobulin preparations. Use of these testing kits in combination with use of products containing nonglucose sugars can result in a falsely elevated POCT glucose value. The US Food and Drug Administration (FDA) has released a Public Health Notification that provides a list of GDH-PQQ glucose test strips; this can be accessed at http://www.fda.gov/MedicalDevices/Safety/AlertsandNotices/PublicHealthNotifications/. In cases where it is not possible to avoid test strips that contain GDH-PQQ, errors can be avoided by use of plasma glucose. This is particularly important for elevated glucose values or those that are inconsistent with a patient's history or glucose pattern.
- Hematocrit level can affect the precision of POCT glucose: A low hematocrit can result in a falsely high glucose reading, whereas a high hematocrit can result in a falsely low reading. These readings should be confirmed with plasma glucose.

Urinary Glucose

Urinary glucose is a semi-quantitative measurement of glycosuria, which represents hyperglycemia above the renal threshold, that is, plasma glucose around 180 mg/dL (10 mmol/L) in many patients. The renal threshold can differ significantly with the duration of a patient's diabetes as well as average glucose levels. Prior to the advent of widely available portable glucose meters, urinary glucose was used for home monitoring. Currently, urinary glucose rarely is used for outpatients, and it is not useful for hospitalized patients.

Glycated Proteins: Hemoglobin A_{1C} and Fructosamine

Hemoglobin A_{1C}

The A_{1C} is a measure of glycosylation of the hemoglobin molecule, which occurs as a nonenzymatic process over time. In patients with diabetes, glycosylation rates rise, reflecting the increased ambient blood glucose levels. Because the average lifetime of a red blood cell is approximately 120 days, the A_{1C} measurement reflects average glucose concentration for that period of time, although weighted toward more recent trends. The relationship between the A_{1C} value and estimated average glucose has been prospectively investigated and can be defined by the following equation: average glucose (mg/dL) $= 28.7 \times A_{1C} - 46.7$. Alternatively, a calculator is available at http://professional.diabetes.org/eAG.

The A_{1C} is the gold standard for assessment of glycemic control, with the ADA targeting A_{1C} levels below 7% as the therapeutic goal for most patients. As of 2010, the A_{1C} has been recommended by the International Expert Committee for screening and diagnostic purposes, with a level of at least 6.5% diagnostic of diabetes. A level of 5.7–6.5% represents "at risk" for diabetes, although this is not the same as a diagnosis of prediabetes made by a glucose-based test.

The A_{1C} is a useful test in hospitalized patients, both for diagnostic purposes and to gather objective information about recent glycemic control. Exceptions include patients who have cause for inaccurate A_{1C} (as below), as well as those who have an outpatient A_{1C} value documented in the prior 30 days.

Conditions Causing Inaccurate A_{1C} Readings

A longstanding concern about use of A_{1C} was the lack of standardization among various methods at different institutions. However, the A_{1C} assay methods have now been largely standardized; most laboratories now use the high-performance liquid chromatographic technique. The following conditions are some of the more common causes of inaccurate A_{1C}; other, rarer conditions also may affect the measurement.

- Recent blood transfusion: dilutes the patient's red cells with those of the donor and will give a falsely low A_{1C}.
- Anemia, including hemolytic anemia, symptomatic β-thalassemia, and sickle cell anemia: Any condition that results in an overall increased rate of red cell turnover can result in a falsely low A_{1C}. Conversely, iron deficiency anemia or other

conditions that result in a decreased rate of red cell production can result in a falsely elevated A_{1C}.

- Pregnancy: In early pregnancy, fetal red cell production can lower the A_{1C} level. Later in pregnancy, increased red cell turnover lowers the normal range for A_{1C}.
- Splenectomy: the resulting decreased red cell destruction can result in higher A_{1C} levels.

Point-of-Care A_{1C}

Point-of-care A_{1C} measurement is performed using a capillary blood sample. In an office-based setting, its use has been observed to result in more frequent intensification of diabetes regimens as well as small but significant improvements in A_{1C} of 0.1–0.5%. Point-of-care A_{1C} testing (via the DCA 2000 model) appears to measure slightly different values than from plasma A_{1C} testing, although by no more than 0.5%. There may also be slightly more intra- and interindividual variability. Newer POC instruments are now available, and although more studies are needed to confirm reliability with standardized assays, the POC method seems promising for convenient monitoring of glucose control in outpatients. There are no data for use of point-of-care A_{1C} testing in the inpatient setting, and its use is not recommended currently.

Fructosamine

Fructosamine is a glycated serum protein that is formed as the result of a reaction between glucose and albumin. Its serum concentration also can be used to estimate glycemia, and there is generally a good correlation between serum fructosamine and A_{1C}. However, routine clinical use of fructosamine is limited by several factors. First, fructosamine only reflects glycemia for the prior 2–3 weeks, as opposed to A_{1C}, which reflects 2–3 months. Second, fructosamine can show considerable variability, even within a single patient, which makes successive measurements more difficult to interpret. Finally, fructosamine level correlates with serum albumin level, and appropriate adjustments must be made for patients with hypoalbuminemia. Overall, the clinical utility of fructosamine is limited, and use in the inpatient setting is not recommended.

Insulin, Pro-insulin, and C-Peptide

Insulin production in the β-cell is a multistep process. Its direct precursor is a molecule called pro-insulin, which is comprised of two components: (1) the future insulin molecule, and (2) 31 amino acids of the "connecting peptide," or

C-peptide. During the final phase of production, insulin is cleaved from the C-peptide, and both are packaged into secretory granules for release into circulation. Pro-insulin and C-peptide are not thought to play a significant independent role in glucose homeostasis, but they are useful as plasma markers of endogenous insulin production.

Likewise, insulin precursor measurements are not useful for evaluation of inpatients with diabetes. The C-peptide level can be useful in diabetic patients who are relatively stable on treatment; in this setting, the C-peptide value, in combination with history, physical examination, and antibody levels, can be used to make the distinction between type 1 and type 2 diabetes. In acute illness, however, insulin and insulin precursor measurements often are inaccurate. In patients presenting with severe hyperglycemia, a low C-peptide level may represent either a true absence of endogenous insulin, as in type 1 diabetes, or the physiologic result of hyperglycemia and glucose toxicity in type 2 diabetes. Conversely, a normal level may be present in a patient with insulin resistance and type 2 diabetes or in a patient with early type 1 diabetes in the honeymoon phase (i.e., that has not yet had full destruction of pancreatic β-cells). Use of the C-peptide level as a guide for initial therapy in patients with type 2 diabetes has not been shown to lead to better glycemic control.

Markers of endogenous insulin production are useful in hospitalized patients who are undergoing evaluation for fasting hypoglycemia, which should be done in collaboration with an endocrinology consultant.

Insulin measurement sometimes is undertaken as a measure of insulin resistance. However, this generally is thought to be unreliable because of high inter- and intraindividual variability. Research studies often use a measure called the homeostatic model assessment (HOMA) for β-cell function or insulin resistance, but this is not useful for inpatient management.

Autoantibody Markers

Type 1 diabetes is an autoimmune disease, characterized by T cell-mediated destruction of the pancreatic β-cell. Autoantibodies have been detected in up to 90% of patients with immune-mediated diabetes. There are three categories of autoantibodies: (1) antibodies to insulin, (2) antibodies to the islet cell and its antigens (glutamate decarboxylase 65 [GAD], tyrosine phosphatase-related proteins islet antigen 2 [IA-2A/ICA 512], and IA-2β) and (3) antibodies to the insulin secretory apparatus. The zinc transporter antibody ZnT8 was recently identified as an autoantigen in this group.

Autoantibody testing to evaluate for type 1 diabetes is relatively specific but somewhat insensitive, partly because the levels may decline over time in patients with longstanding disease. Furthermore, autoantibody testing is expensive and, in most cases, does not add information beyond the clinical impressions of the provider. Overall, the presence of autoantibodies is supportive, but not required, for a diagnosis of type 1 diabetes mellitus.

Ketones

Serum Ketones

Production of ketone bodies is a normal response to the body's shortage of glucose during starvation, and is meant to provide an alternate source of fuel via free fatty acids. Insulin deficiency and subsequent perceived shortage of glucose, as in diabetic ketoacidosis (DKA), provokes lipolysis, producing free fatty acids. The fatty acids are then transferred to the liver, where they are oxidized to become ketone bodies. In DKA, the ketone β-hydroxybutyrate increases to a great extent, disproportionately to the other ketones, acetone and acetoacetate.

The test strips for measurement of serum ketones do not capture β-hydroxybutyrate, but they strongly capture acetoacetate and acetone. Despite the physiologic predominance of β-hydroxybutyrate, this method usually is sufficient for ketone detection during DKA. However, occasional serum ketone tests may be read as negative even in the presence of true DKA. A specific β-hydroxybutyrate level is available in some laboratories, but it is rarely necessary to confirm the diagnosis. To avoid confusion, serum ketone levels should be ordered in combination with electrolytes, arterial blood gas, and other appropriate laboratory assessments and should be interpreted in the context of the clinical presentation. Further information about diagnosis and management of DKA can be found in Chapter 6: Hyperglycemic Emergencies.

During treatment with insulin and fluids, β-hydroxybutyrate is oxidized to acetoacetate and acetone, which can result in persistent elevation of measured serum ketone levels, despite obvious clinical improvement. For this reason, serial serum ketone measurements are not recommended for routine monitoring during DKA management.

Urine Ketones

The urine ketone measurement represents a semi-quantitative level of acetone and acetoacetate, with a positive test indicating ketoacidosis. The primary advantage of the urine measurement over the serum measurement is that it will be positive prior to presence of measurable ketones in the serum. Therefore, it is a quick and easy way to screen for DKA in patients with hyperglycemia. However, as with other laboratory tests in diabetes, the presence of urine ketones alone is not definitive and must be interpreted in the context of the overall clinical picture, serum electrolytes, anion gap, and serum ketone measurement.

Urine Microalbumin

The urine microalbumin measurement represents small but abnormal amounts of albuminuria, present in early stages of diabetic nephropathy, prior to the development of frank proteinuria and nephrotic syndrome (Table 4.2). Additionally, the

Table 4.2 American Diabetes Association definitions for levels of albuminuria in patients with diabetes

	Volume of albumin excretion		
	mg/24 h	mcg/min	mcg/mg of creatinine
Normal	<30	<20	<30
Microalbuminuria	30–300	20–200	30–300
Clinical albuminuria	>300	>200	>300

presence of microalbuminuria in patients with diabetes is a predictor of ischemic cardiovascular (CV) events related to the development of atherosclerosis.

Urine microalbumin is not specific to diabetic nephropathy; in fact, there are multiple causes for albuminuria in a hospitalized patient. Because microalbuminuria related to other causes can be transient, it is best to assess urine microalbumin in outpatients who are in stable condition. Even in the outpatient setting, the ADA recommends confirmation of multiple measurements over a period of months before making the diagnosis of diabetic nephropathy. If microalbuminuria is identified, it is important to consider other possible causes, such as

- Urinary tract infection
- Severe hyperglycemia
- Acute febrile illness
- Heart failure
- Hypertension
- Strenuous exercise in the last 24 h
- Pregnancy

Cardiovascular Risk Assessment

Lipid Profile

Serum lipid levels are a well-characterized component of cardiovascular (CV) risk, and their measurement is useful both for risk prediction and assessment of the effectiveness of a patient's lipid-lowering therapy. The ADA recommends an annual screening fasting lipid profile for all patients with type 2 diabetes. Furthermore, the National Cholesterol Education Program Adult Treatment Panel (ATP) III suggested use of statins and dietary therapy in all patients with diabetes, even for those without known CV disease (CVD), because of their poor prognosis once CVD becomes manifest. Therapeutic goals are based on ATP III recommendations for levels of low-density lipoprotein (LDL); these have gained support from more recent data, including the Heart Protection Study (HPS). For patients with diabetes and without known CVD, the risk for future events is roughly equivalent to those in the opposite situation—without diabetes but with history of CVD. HPS data for this population support the ATP-III recommended LDL goal of no more than 100 mg/dL

(2.5 mmol/L). Patients with both diabetes and history of CVD are at very high risk for future cardiac events and, in the HPS, obtained the greatest benefit from lipid-lowering therapy with statins. For these patients, it is reasonable to attempt to achieve a very low LDL level of 70 mg/dL (1.8 mmol/L) or less.

Although lipid panels frequently are ordered for patients in the hospital and can be useful, their reliability is limited; conditions such as acute myocardial infarction and systemic inflammation may cause falsely low readings.

High-Sensitivity C-Reactive Protein (hsCRP)

C-reactive protein (CRP) is an acute-phase inflammatory protein that is released from hepatocytes in response to acute injury, infection, or other inflammatory stimuli. An increase in total CRP is expected in association with many conditions requiring hospitalization. Increased CRP can be seen on a subtle level in diseases with long-term, low-grade inflammation, such as atherosclerotic disease. Traditional CRP assays have had limited analytical sensitivity, with a minimum detectable level of 0.5–1 mg/dL, and were not useful for evaluating these slight levels of inflammation. However, new high-sensitivity assays, like the rate nephelometry method, can detect CRP concentrations as low as 0.02 mg/dL. These high-sensitivity CRP (hsCRP) assays have become widely available for clinical use. This availability, combined with the short half-life (about 18 h), the stability of CRP in serum (lasts up to 3 days at room temperature), and evidence for its correlation with atherosclerotic disease have made this a popular test for CV risk stratification. Furthermore, in patients with type 2 diabetes, there may be an independent association between hsCRP levels greater than 0.3 mg/dL and risk for death from CVD. Finally, data from the JUPITER (Justification for the Use of Statins in Prevention: an Interventional Trial Evaluating Rosuvastatin) trial suggests that use of rosuvastatin in patients with normal LDL cholesterol but elevated hsCRP may provide CV risk protection. For these reasons, hsCRP may be a useful test in the outpatient setting; however, the utility of this test in hospitalized patients, especially those with infection or inflammation from other conditions, is limited.

Bibliography

American Diabetes Association. Standards of medical care in diabetes—2010. *Diabetes Care.* 2010;33(suppl 1):S11–S61.

Beaser RS. *Joslin's Diabetes Deskbook. A Guide for Primary Care Providers.* 2nd ed. Boston, MA: Joslin Diabetes Center; 2008.

Bingley PJ. Clinical applications of diabetes antibody testing. *J Clin Endocrinol Metab.* 2010;95(1):25–33.

Camacho P, Gharib H, Sizemore G. *Evidence-Based Endocrinology.* 2nd ed. Philadelphia, PA: Lippincott Williams & Wilkins; 2007.

Expert Committee on the Diagnosis and Classification of Diabetes Mellitus. Report of the Expert Committee on the Diagnosis and Classification of Diabetes Mellitus. *Diabetes Care.* 1997;20(7):1183–1197.

Expert Panel on Detection, Evaluation, and Treatment of High Blood Cholesterol in Adults. Executive Summary of the Third Report of the National Cholesterol Education Program (NCEP)

Expert Panel on Detection, Evaluation, and Treatment of High Blood Cholesterol in Adults (Adult Treatment Panel III). *JAMA*. 2001;285(19):2486–2497.

Grundy SM, Cleeman JI, Bairey Merz CM, et al. for the Coordinating Committee of the National Cholesterol Education Program. Implications of recent clinical trials for the National Cholesterol Education Program Adult Treatment Panel III Guidelines. *Circulation*. 2004;110(2):227–239.

Heart Protection Study Collaborative Group. MRC/BHF Heart Protection Study of cholesterol lowering with simvastatin in 20,536 high-risk individuals: a randomised placebo-controlled trial. *Lancet*. 2002;360(9326):7–22.

International Expert Committee. International Expert Committee report on the role of the A_{1C} assay in the diagnosis of diabetes. *Diabetes Care*. 2009;32(12):1–8.

Karon BS, Griesmann L, Scott R, et al. Evaluation of the impact of hematocrit and other interference on the accuracy of hospital-based glucose meters. *Diabetes Technol Ther.*, 2008;10(2):111–120.

Khan AI, Vasquez Y, Gray J, Wians FH Jr, Kroll MH. The variability of results between point-of-care testing glucose meters and the central laboratory analyzer. *Arch Pathol Lab Med*. 2006;130(10):1527–1537.

Khosla N, Sarafidis PA, Bakris GL. Microalbuminuria. *Clin Lab Med*. 2006;26(3):635–653.

Matthews DR, Hosker JP, Rudenski AS, Naylor BA, Treacher DF, Turner RC. Homeostasis model assessment: insulin resistance and beta-cell function from fasting plasma glucose and insulin concentrations in man. *Diabetologia*. 1985;28(7):412–419.

Miller CD, Barnes CS, Phillips LS, Ziemer DC, Gallina DL, Cook CB, et al. Rapid A_{1c} availability improves clinical decision-making in an urban primary care clinic. *Diabetes Care*. 2003;26(4):1158–1163.

Nathan DM, Kuenen J, Borg R, Zheng H, Schoenfeld D, Heine RJ, A1c-Derived Average Glucose Study Group. Translating the A1C assay into estimated average glucose values. *Diabetes Care*. 2008;31(8):1473–1478.

National Glycated Hemoglobin Standardization Project. http://www.ngsp.org/prog/index.html. Accessed May 10, 2009.

Ridker PM, Danielson E, Fonseca FA, JUPITER Study Group. Rosuvastatin to prevent vascular events in men and women with elevated C-reactive protein. *N Engl J Med*. 2008;359(21):2195–2207.

Sacks DB, Bruns DE, Goldstein DE, et al. Guidelines and recommendations for laboratory analysis in the diagnosis and management of diabetes mellitus. *Clin Chem*. 2002;48(3):436–472.

Soinio M, Marniemi J, Laakso M, et al. High-sensitivity C-reactive protein and coronary heart disease mortality in patients with type 2 diabetes. A 7-year follow-up study. *Diabetes Care*. 2006;29(2):329–333.

Tamborlane WV, Kollman C, Steffes MW, Ruedy KJ, Dongyuan X, Beck RW, et al. The Diabetes Research in Children Network Study Group. Comparison of fingerstick hemoglobin A1c levels assayed by DCA 2000 with the DCCT/EDIC central laboratory assay: results of a Diabetes Research in Children Network (DirecNet) Study. *Pediatr Diabetes*, 2005;6(1):13–16.

Wilson AM, Ryan MC, Boyle AJ. The novel role of C-reactive protein in cardiovascular disease: Risk marker or pathogen. *Int J Cardiol*. 2006;106(3):291–297.

Chapter 5
Inpatient Diabetes Education: Realistic and Evidence-Based

Ellen D. Davis, Anne T. Nettles, and Ashley Leak

Keywords Diabetes education · Diabetes self-care · Patient-centered approach · Empathetic listening · Multidisciplinary teamwork · Teachable moment

Hospitalization can present an opportunity to address unique urgent learning needs. Although some would argue that the hospital is a poor setting for patient education, this does not have to be the case. Brief targeted diabetes education is readily available, and take-home materials can reinforce instruction. Given the sheer volume of inpatients with diabetes, dedicated resources for their care and education are essential.

Inpatients with well-controlled diabetes sometimes find hospitalization a loss of personal control filled with challenges. Other inpatients may never have been able to achieve good blood glucose control, and still others may not even know that they have diabetes. Recent studies have shown that providers have a tendency to neglect diabetes and hyperglycemia in the hospital, which leads to missed opportunities for teaching. In this chapter, we discuss these opportunities and how providers can best equip individuals for self-care after discharge.

Understanding Diabetes Education

Why Do Patients Need Diabetes Education?

Self-care education results in the following:

- An improvement in the patient's ability to problem-solve at home.
- Better glycemic control.
- Improved quality of life.

E.D. Davis (✉)
Department of Advanced Clinical Practice, Duke University Hospital, Durham, NC 27710, USA;
Duke University School of Nursing, Durham, NC 27710, USA
e-mail: davis010@mc.duke.edu

L.F. Lien et al. (eds.), *Glycemic Control in the Hospitalized Patient*,
DOI 10.1007/978-1-60761-006-9_5, © Springer Science+Business Media, LLC 2011

Why Do Patients Need Diabetes Education in the Hospital?

It is often the case that patients are not well informed about diabetes self-care because comprehensive outpatient diabetes education may not be convenient or even available to them.

What Factors Interfere with Inpatient Diabetes Education?

There are a variety of factors that interfere with effective inpatient diabetes education. In the busy inpatient setting, patients may not be interested or engaged in educational efforts, physical condition, literacy, numeracy, culture, mental health, and finances influence knowledge, learning, and self-care possibilities. Additionally, there are many misconceptions about diabetes, at both the provider and patient levels. Provider misconceptions include the following:

- Diabetes care and education are only outpatient issues.
- Every adverse patient outcome is a result of poor self-care.
- When people get diabetes, they do not mind suddenly making major lifestyle changes.
- Scare tactics motivate patients to make lifestyle changes. "If you don't do what I (the 'expert') say, you'll go blind or have your feet amputated."
- Handouts about diabetes and a few "discharge orders" are all that patients need.
- Physicians don't have time to effectively support their patients.
- When providers use the word "stress," patients know what it means. Although providers usually are referring to physiological stress, patients interpret this term as meaning that they are doing something wrong by not handling their emotional stress well.
- Diabetes self-care is the only thing patients have on their minds.

Patient misconceptions include

- Chronic complications are inevitable, so self-care is a waste of time.
- "Pills worked before, so I shouldn't need insulin."
- "I'm 'guilty' of bringing this on myself." ("My spirits are low and I can't do all of these things they want me to do.")
- "Needing insulin is a sign that I, and the treatment, have 'failed'."
- "I have to deprive myself by eating 'diabetic food'."

  - "I will be hungry all the time."
  - "It's all about not eating 'sugar' and about eating 'special foods'."

There are specific tactics clinicians can use when dealing with patient misconceptions, while also effectively imparting information:

- Use nonjudgmental language.
- Avoid negative words:

  - Noncompliant. The use of *noncompliant* is believed by diabetes education experts to negatively affect patient outcomes.
  - Failure (i.e., "diet failure" or "oral agent failure"). Progression to need for oral medication or insulin may be viewed by the patient as a personal failure or serious character flaw. People are not motivated when they perceive themselves as failures, and people do not act on both negative and positive associations at the same time.
  - Bad blood sugars. Use "safe" or "unsafe."
  - Sliding scale insulin. Many patients infer, "Don't take insulin unless your blood sugar is high." When describing correction bolus or supplements for scheduled insulin, point out the difference and probable need for later, proactive scheduled insulin adjustments.

- Use *patient-centered approaches.* Starting with the patient's agenda produces the best outcomes. For example, if the patient is concerned about nocturnal hypoglycemia, start by collaboratively discussing prevention, recognition, and treatment of hypoglycemia.

  - This type of lifestyle coaching, as part of a larger lifestyle intervention, resulted in improved glycemic levels in the Diabetes Prevention Program (DPP, 2002) and all ensuing community-based trials of lifestyle interventions. The Diabetes Control and Complication Trial (DCCT, 1994) also produced outstanding glycemic results with significantly decreased complications through patient-centered education with individualized problem solving.

- Elicit patient candor through *empathetic listening.* If possible, sit down and establish direct eye contact with the patient. Acknowledge the patient's individual concerns. (Patients are not interested in "diabetes," but in their own lives.)
- *Ask specific but open-ended questions* rather than lecturing. Evidence shows that this takes less time than repeatedly listing what every person "should" do.

  - "What are you most worried about when it comes to taking care of your diabetes?" The answer may reflect cultural misunderstandings that may be dealt with easily, like, "I can't afford 'diabetic' food."
  - Rather than saying, "Follow this list of instructions," ask, "What one thing will you do differently when you go home or until your next outpatient visit?"
  - "On a scale of 1–10, how would you rate the way you eat for your diabetes?" "What one thing could you do when you go home to make that upward move you mentioned?"
  - Rather than say, "Get more exercise," ask, "At what time of day could you take a walk and with whom?"
  - Asking, "Do you have any questions?" after provider-centered care seldom elicits information that helps provider improve patient outcomes.

- Provide up-to-date resources: on-demand patient educational TV, written materials, translation services, patient teaching by staff nurses, diabetes resource nurses or champions, and clinical nurse specialists. Many hospitals have resources like these; find out what is available to you, and use it!

Key Points: Education Strategy

- Human beings change one behavior at a time.
- Asking good questions and listening are keys to all patient interaction.
- People respond more positively to compliments for what they are doing well rather than to criticism or lectures on what is needed for improvements.
- "Covering the material" and "rules are rules" patient education approaches do not improve glycemic control or quality of life or reduce costs for systems.
- Behavioral change strategies (like those listed above) work better than lectures and "should" talk. No one feels upbeat enough to make continuous major lifestyle changes when feeling judged, blamed, guilty, or terrified of the future.
- A good first question to ask patients is "What have you heard about taking care of diabetes?"

The Content of Diabetes Education

The American Diabetes Association (ADA) 2010 Standards of Medical Care suggest that a smooth transition to home be ensured by anticipation of the post-discharge regimen, effects of the current illness on glycemic control, and, for those with hyperglycemia only, follow-up diagnostic testing for diabetes. There is comprehensive ADA diabetes education curricula designed for outpatients, but in the hospital, the ADA prefers a more focused, "survival skills" approach. Two useful education constructs, which are described in detail below, are the following: (1) The American Association of Diabetes Educators (AADE) AADE7™ Self-Care Behaviors and (2) a synthesis of The Joint Commission, AADE, ADA, and other groups' published pre-discharge assessment and education content.

AADE7™ Self-Care Behaviors

The AADE believes that behavior change can be most successfully achieved when patients follow seven self-care behaviors:

1. *Healthy eating* today means healthy foods in reasonable portions to meet weight and nutrition goals. Individual strategies for eating less, if overweight, and eating breakfast daily are top counseling priorities. If the patient is taking insulin, spreading the carbohydrate foods across the day requires extra attention. Referral for nutrition counseling is appropriate at discharge if needed.
2. *Being active* is the same for patients with diabetes as for the general public: Patients should aim for at least 150 min of physical exercise a week, like walking, each day with resistance training three times/week. Main point: Get started.

3. *Glucose monitoring* is a frequent occurrence for hospitalized patients. Bedside glucose testing poses a "teachable moment" for staff nurses. (See section, "What Can Nurses Do?")

4. *Medications* may change from oral agents to insulin while the patient is in the hospital. Although this can alarm some patients, many are relieved to find that injections are not as bad as they had feared. Insulin initiation can be explained as merely a reliable way to rapidly control glucose during acute illness. In helping patients deal with taking insulin at home, ask them about their concerns, and then provide information. When insulin is new, prevention, recognition, and treatment of hypoglycemia must be discussed.

5. *Problem solving* is a common method learned by healthcare professionals, and is rarely formally familiar to patients. When they learn to address self-care problems systematically and objectively, they can be more successful. It is helpful to explain this approach as a 6-step process.

   1. Identify the problem objectively and specifically.
   2. Consider a variety of possible strategies to address the problem.
   3. Consider the pros and cons of each strategy.
   4. Pick the best strategy.
   5. Try it, and evaluate how it is working.
   6. If the problem is not solved, identify barriers and try to reduce them or try another strategy.

   More than 99% of patient outcomes are the result of patient problem solving at home. Some problems have no solutions; for example, the disease will not be cured. For unsolvable problems, patients need to use enhanced coping mechanisms (below).

6. *Reducing risks* includes regular screening for complications and comorbidities. Patients should be advised that there are a variety of ways to understand how diabetes affects the body, including the hemoglobin A_{1C} level, foot examination, urine microalbumin screening, dilated eye exams, and dental exams. Patients can discuss these screening tests with their outpatient provider.

7. *Healthy coping* is essential in daily diabetes life; it is about decision making and performing self-care. Self-care is challenging for most people because diabetes care involves daily disruptions of the usual. Interestingly, social support has been found to be one of the most helpful self-care strategies. Providers should routinely assess sources of support and provide information about other resources in the community. A wide variety of coping tactics have been used, such as relaxation, guided imagery, humor, music, and exercise. The strategies are different for different people.

Synthesis of Published Recommendations for Assessments and Education during Discharge Planning

- Assess current practice of self-care and provide needed information on basic diabetes self-management skills for newly diagnosed patients and others with changes in the regimen, using focused, short sessions. Does the patient require outpatient diabetes self-management education?

- Does the patient prepare his or her own meals? Discuss consistent eating patterns. Advise the patient to avoid concentrated sugar foods until he or she has ongoing counseling by a diabetes educator on how to do so safely.
- Can the patient perform self-monitoring of blood glucose at a reasonable frequency? List resources for home blood glucose monitoring and sharing of results with the healthcare provider. Can the patient teach-back (verbalize what he or she understood) that sharing home testing numbers results in improved medical care? If relevant, the patient should do a demonstration at least once.
- Can the patient take his or her diabetes medications or insulin accurately? The patient should demonstrate drawing up and self-administering insulin at least once or twice. Is there a family member who can assist with tasks that the patient cannot perform? Is a home health nurse needed to facilitate transition to the home?
- Explore possibilities for individualized exercise.
- Provide information on prevention, symptoms, and treatment of hypoglycemia.
- Provide information on hyperglycemia and "Sick Day Rules," since not understanding that insulin is needed with hyperglycemia even if unable to eat, causes many hospitalizations.
- Help patients understand who and when to call for help and specific arrangements for follow-up, including appointments for outpatient diabetes education in hospitals, physicians' offices, communities, churches, senior centers, health departments, and others.

Every Patient Is Unique

Consider the following scenarios:

- A 30-year-old man with type 1 diabetes admitted with diabetic ketoacidosis: Information should focus on the diabetic crisis and any deficient self-care skills.
- A 20-year-old woman with a hemoglobin A_{1C} of 11%, who has not been informed about the consequences of an unplanned pregnancy and diabetes, needs preconceptual diabetes counseling first.

Who Are the Educators?

Inpatient education requires multidisciplinary teamwork. Patients learn about chronic disease management at each encounter with healthcare providers. Providing patient-centered education and support cannot be delayed until the discharge day! It must be effectively implemented, starting with an admission assessment.

Role of Physician and Other Providers

- Diagnosis and medical decision making.
- Communication with other providers.
- Use teachable moments with patients each day. For example, when seeing a patient with diabetes who is drinking fruit juice and eating pancakes for breakfast, use this as an opportunity to talk about the effect of carbohydrates on glucose levels, realizing that appropriate carbohydrate foods are needed. Realize that patients may be afraid to eat and may make choices based on out-of-date admonishments, like, "Don't eat sugar." When a patient asks how often to test, listen, reflect and collaboratively design an achievable plan, like staggered or paired testing.
- When a patient needs to start on daily insulin for home use and says he or she is strongly opposed to doing so, the provider can say, "Will you tell us more about your thinking regarding taking insulin at home?" Then, empathetically help patients look at risk–benefit issues. After this nonjudgmental discussion, usually patients decide that home insulin is a beneficial, achievable part of their future, and perhaps, short-term, self-care.
- When talking with patients about home blood glucose testing, remember that their particular insurance coverage of the strips used for testing is the main factor in choice of meter and frequency of testing.

Role of Staff Nurse

- Assess and supplement the basic knowledge and skills of people with diabetes. Listen, explain, and teach discharge recommendations.
- If registered nurses do glucose monitoring, they can assess the patient's use of self-monitoring of blood glucose, the frequency of home testing, and strategy for sharing of results with the outpatient provider. During individualized education, discuss meaningful home testing; for example, staggered time schedules can be cost effective. A second strategy is to test once a day in a "pair," like before and after exercise or before and 2 h after a meal.
- Inpatient-type education also can be provided in emergency departments. Outpatient education referral is essential.
- Assess sources of social support and provide information about other resources in the community.
- If a hospital is closely linked to an ADA- or AADE-recognized outpatient education program, inpatient and outpatient nurses can collaborate, document on the same educational forms, and share teaching responsibilities to enhance the patient's experience and eliminate duplication.

Role of the Certified Diabetes Educator (CDE), Nurse, and Dietician

- The role of the CDE in the inpatient setting is to serve as a resource and role model for other healthcare professionals.

- The CDE also can provide direct patient education for patients with complex medical problems.

Training and Support for Healthcare Providers Engaged in Diabetes Inpatient Education

Training is needed for providers to educate inpatients with diabetes. Numerous approaches can be useful: publications, unit-based classes, mentoring, online programs, rounds with diabetes care providers, clinical nurse specialists and discharge planners, and individual unit diabetes nurse champions.

Key Points: Inpatient Diabetes Education

- Acknowledge that all healthcare providers support and educate patients toward better outcomes.
- Listen to the patient and collaborate to develop a plan.
- Address the most crucial education concepts and practices, including healthy diet, activity plan, medication administration, blood glucose monitoring, and sharing of results, hypoglycemia, hyperglycemia, and managing minor illness, emergency care, and plans for follow-up.
- Practice behavioral change strategies, like motivational Interviewing, which take less healthcare provider-time and produce improved outcomes.

Bibliography

American Association of Diabetes Educators (AADE). AADE7™ Self Care Behaviors. Measurable behavior change is the desired outcome of diabetes education. http://www.diabeteseducator.org/ProfessionalResources/AADE7/. Accessed April 9, 2009.

American Association of Diabetes Educator (AADE). Inpatient position statement. http://www.diabeteseducator.org/ProfessionalResources/. Accessed April 9, 2009.

American Diabetes Association. National standards for diabetes self-management education. http://care.diabetesjournals.org/content/33/Supplement_1/. Accessed March16, 2010.

Anderson BJ, Rubin RR. Practical Psychology for Diabetes Clinicians. Alexandria, VA: American Diabetes Association; 2002.

Anderson RM, Funnell MM, Burkhart N, Gillard ML, Nwankwo R. 101 Tips for Behavior Change in Diabetes Education. Alexandria, VA: American Diabetes Association; 2002.

Cochran J, Conn VS. Meta-analysis of quality of life outcomes following diabetes self-management training. Diabetes Educ. 2008;34(5):815–823.

Clement S, Braithwaite S, Magee MF, et al. Management of diabetes and hyperglycemia in hospitals. Diabetes Care. 2004;27(2):553–591.

Davis E, Vander Meer J, Yarborough P, Roth S. Using solution-focused therapy strategies in empowerment-based education. Diabetes Educ. 1999;25:249–257.

Davis E, White A, Muro T. Diabetes education in the emergency department: another challenge. American Association of Diabetes Educators On-line Article Archive. http://www.diabeteseducator.org/ProfessionalResources/Periodicals/Practice/ Online Archive. Accessed April 9, 2009.

Delahanty LM, Nathan DM. Implications of the diabetes prevention program and Look AHEAD clinical trials for lifestyle interventions. *J Am Diet Assoc.* 2008;108(suppl 4):S66–S72.

Duncan I, Birkmeyer C, Coughlin S, Li Q, Sherr D, Boren S. Assessing the value of education. *Diabetes Educ.* 2009;35(5):752–760.

Funnell M, Brown TL, Childs BP, Haas LB, Hosey GM, Jensen B, et al. National standards for diabetes self management education. *Diabetes Care.* 2010;33(suppl 1):S89–S96.

Jackson L. Translating the Diabetes Prevention Program into Practice: a review of community interventions. *Diabetes Educ.* 2009;35(2):309–320.

Leak A, Davis ED, Mabrey M, Houchin L. Diabetes self management and patient education in hospitalized oncology patients. *Clin J Oncol Nurs.* 2009;13(2): 205–210.

Levinson W, Gorawara-Bhat R, Lamb J. A study of patient clues and physician responses in primary care and surgical settings. *JAMA.* 2000;284(8):1021–1027.

Manchester C. Diabetes education in the hospital: establishing professional competency. *Diabetes Spectr.* 2008;21:268–271.

Nettles AT. Patient education in the hospital. *Diabetes Spectr.* 2005;18(1):44–48.

Parkin C, Hinnen D, Campbell K, Geil P, Tetrick D, Polonsky W. Effective use of paired testing in type 2 diabetes: practical applications in clinical practice. *Diabetes Educ.* 2009;35(6):915–927.

Rollnick S, Miller W, Butler C. *Motivational Interviewing in Health Care: Helping Patients Change Behavior.* New York, NY: Guilford Press; 2008.

Turek P, Mueller M, Egede L. Estimating physician effects on glycemic control in the treatment of diabetes: methods, effects sizes, and implications for treatment policy. *Diabetes Care.* 2008;31(5):869–873.

Urbanski P, Wolf A, Herman WH. Cost-effectiveness of diabetes education. *J Am Diet Assoc.* 2008;108(suppl 4):S6–S11.

Welch G, Rose G, Ernst D. Motivational interviewing and diabetes: what is it, how is it used, and does it work? *Diabetes Spectr.* 2006;19:5–11.

Chapter 6
Hyperglycemic Emergencies: Diabetic Ketoacidosis and Hyperosmolar Hyperglycemic State

Leonor Corsino and Lekshmi T. Nair

Keywords Diabetic ketoacidosis · Hyperosmolar nonketotic hyperglycemia · Counterregulatory hormones · Ketosis · Acidosis · IV insulin

Diabetic Ketoacidosis

Diabetic ketoacidosis (DKA) is a serious acute complication of type 1 diabetes mellitus and, less commonly, type 2 diabetes mellitus. DKA continues to be an important cause of morbidity and mortality in individuals with diabetes, despite significant advances in the treatment of DKA. With prompt and appropriate treatment, the mortality is rated between 5–20%, but this increases substantially with aging and the presence of concomitant severe illness.

Case Presentation

A 32-year-old woman presented to the emergency department complaining of nausea, vomiting, and abdominal pain for the last 24 h.[1] According to the patient, she was in her usual state of health until 1 week prior to presentation when she developed a cough with chills and fevers. Over the next few days, her condition progressed to include nausea, vomiting, and mid-epigastric pain. She denied any prior medical conditions and stated that she had always been healthy. Upon arrival at the emergency department, she was an alert and oriented, young, obese, black woman. Her blood pressure was 116/73 mmHg, pulse was 114 beats/min, respiratory rate was 20 breaths/min, and temperature was 100°F. Pertinent physical exam findings were decreased breath sounds in the right lower lung and mid-epigastric tenderness.

L. Corsino (✉)
Division of Endocrinology, Metabolism, and Nutrition, Department of Medicine, Duke University Medical Center, Durham, NC 27710, USA
e-mail: corsi002@mc.duke.edu

[1]The case presented above does not represent a real patient. It was created as an educational aid.

L.F. Lien et al. (eds.), *Glycemic Control in the Hospitalized Patient*,
DOI 10.1007/978-1-60761-006-9_6, © Springer Science+Business Media, LLC 2011

Biochemical evaluation showed the following:

- Sodium: 135 mmol/L [reference: 135–145 mmol/L]
- Potassium: 4 mmol/L [3.5–5.0 mmol/L]
- Chloride: 110 mmol/L [98–108 mmol/L]
- Bicarbonate: 9 mmol/L [21–30 mmol/L]
- Blood urea nitrogen (BUN): 35 mg/dL [7–20 mg/dL]
- Creatinine: 1 mg/dL [0.6–1.3 mg/dL]
- Blood glucose: 550 mg/dL [70–140 mg/dL]
  Blood glucose in mmol/L: (30.5 mmol/L [3.8–7.7 mmol/L])
- Serum osmolality: 313 mOsm/L [277–293 mOsm/L]
- Arterial blood gas: pH: 7.1 [7.35–7.45]
- Urine ketones: positive [negative]

Chest radiography demonstrated right lower lobe pneumonia.

The patient was diagnosed with new-onset diabetes presenting with DKA and right lower lobe pneumonia.

Pathogenesis

DKA is caused by a reduced concentration of circulating insulin with a corresponding increase in counterregulatory hormones, such as glucagon, catecholamines, cortisol, and growth hormone (Fig. 6.1).

Clinical Presentation and Manifestations

Clinical presentation and manifestations include the following:

- Polyuria (increased urination)
- Polydipsia (increased thirst)
- Fatigue
- Weight loss
- Nausea and vomiting
- Abdominal pain, which can resemble an acute abdomen or pancreatitis
- Vital sign abnormalities: tachycardia, tachypnea, hypotension, normo- or hypothermia
- Dry mucous membranes and reduced skin turgor
- Kussmaul breathing (deep and labored breathing pattern often associated with severe metabolic acidosis)
- Mental status changes, including coma
- "Fruity" breath odor, which represents acetone

It should be noted that some patients might present with DKA without prior symptoms or history of diabetes. Also, it is important to understand that DKA per

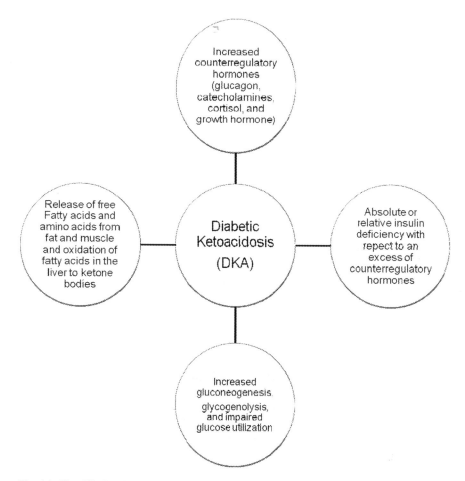

Fig. 6.1 Simplified pathophysiology of diabetic ketoacidosis

se does not cause fever, so the presence of fever may be a clue to the pathogenesis/ precipitating event.

Precipitants

Among precipitants of DKA are

- Infection (the most common)
- New-onset diabetes
- Discontinuation of or inadequate insulin regimen
- Cerebrovascular accidents
- Myocardial infarction
- Alcohol abuse

- Pancreatitis
- Trauma
- Medications (corticosteroids, thiazides, sympathomimetics such as dobutamine and terbutaline)
- Drugs (cocaine)
- Pregnancy
- Psychological problems complicated by eating disorders

Differential Diagnosis

It is critical to remember that most of the information needed to differentiate DKA from other diagnoses will come from a good clinical history.

- Starvation ketosis and alcoholic ketoacidosis: will present with mildly elevated blood glucose (rarely > 200 mg/dL [11.1 mmol/L]) to hypoglycemia; bicarbonate usually not lower than 18 mEq/L.
- Lactic acidosis: Because lactic acidosis is more common in patients with diabetes than in nondiabetic persons and because elevated lactic acid levels may occur in severely volume contracted patients it should always be measured on admission; ketones will not be present.
- Ingestion of drugs (salicylate, methanol, ethylene glycol, isoniazid, and paraldehyde) – these ingestions can be detected on specific drug screens; ethylene glycol can be suggested by the presence of calcium oxalate crystals in the urine; paraldehyde ingestion is indicated by the strong odor on the breath.
- Chronic or acute kidney failure with severe uremia – differentiate by history and biochemical testing.
- There are some case reports of patients with acromegaly presenting with DKA.

Certainly, patients with diabetes also can be affected with the above disorders. These conditions are not mutually exclusive with DKA, and complete evaluation should be conducted in patients who are at risk for multiple-etiology metabolic disturbances.

Evaluation

Urgent evaluation should include the following:

- History and physical examination. The history should focus on possible precipitating factors. Almost 20% of patients presenting to the emergency department with DKA have no previous diagnosis of diabetes.
- Biochemical testing should include plasma glucose, BUN/creatinine, serum and urine ketones, electrolytes (with calculated anion gap), plasma osmolality, urinalysis, complete cell count with differential.
- Chest X- ray, urine, sputum, and blood cultures should also be obtained.

- Calculated anion gap (AG):

  - $AG = [Na^+] - ([Cl^-] + [HCO_3{}^-])$
  - Normal range: 9–12 mmol/L.

- Calculated total plasma osmolality:

  - Total plasma osmolality $= 2 [Na^+ (mmol/L)] + [Glucose (mg/dL)/18] + [BUN (mg/dL)/2.8]$.
  - Normal: 290 ± 5 mOsm/L (this number might have a different range based on each laboratory's reference values).

- Arterial blood gas to evaluate for acidosis.
- Electrocardiogram with attention to signs of hyperkalemia or acute myocardial infarction.

Laboratory Findings

Confirmation of DKA will be completed by presence of anion-gap metabolic acidosis and positive serum and/or urine ketones. Blood glucose almost always will be elevated as well; however, in the case of chronic starvation, blood glucose level may be normal and up to 10% of patients with DKA might present with so-called "euglycemic DKA". Occasionally, serum ketones are read as low or negative because ketone strips, using the nitroprusside reagent, only detect acetoacetate and acetone, while the ketone β(beta) -hydroxybutyrate predominates in DKA. A β (beta) -hydroxybutyrate level is available in some laboratories, but it rarely is necessary to confirm the diagnosis.

Once DKA is confirmed, the patient should be evaluated for precipitating factors. Hemoglobin A_{1C} may be useful to differentiate between poorly controlled or undiagnosed diabetes and an acute event in an otherwise well-controlled patient. Many patients with DKA present with leukocytosis. This is usually proportional to the blood ketone concentrations and might not be indicative of infection. Also, patients with DKA might have elevated lipase, amylase, and liver enzymes. Physicians must always remember that a good clinical history is the key to determine if this is due to pancreatitis or an elevation related to DKA.

Management

Treatment goals include the following:

- Decrease plasma glucose and osmolality by giving IV insulin.
- Increase circulatory volume and perfusion by giving IV fluids.
- Correct electrolyte imbalances. Hyponatremia often will correct with routine management, but potassium and bicarbonate may need to be replaced. In some cases, replacement of phosphorus, calcium, and magnesium may also be required (see section on electrolytes).
- Clear serum and urine ketones.
- Treat precipitating events.

In many cases, intensive care unit (ICU)-level monitoring will be required because of the necessary frequency of monitoring.

Insulin

Prior to initiation of insulin therapy, hypokalemia (less than 3.3 mmol/L) must be treated as detailed under Electrolytes.

Although there are prospective, randomized trial data that support the use of subcutaneous insulin analogs for treatment of uncomplicated DKA, regular insulin given intravenously is still the treatment of choice in the majority of cases.

IV regular insulin is given as follows:

- Therapy should begin with a bolus dose of 0.1–0.15 units/kg of regular IV insulin.
- Along with the bolus dose, a continuous IV insulin infusion is initiated at a rate of 0.1 units/kg/h.
- The goal is an hourly decrease in blood glucose of approximately 50–75 mg/dL (2.75–4.12 mmol/L). Many institutions have an automatic protocol for infusion adjustment based on monitoring results and other parameters. One method for adjustment of the infusion rate can be found in Chapter 3: IV Insulin.
- While the patient is on IV insulin, capillary glucose should be monitored hourly. (Many institutions require ICU status for this intensity of patient care.)
- Continue IV insulin until the patient is stable. The American Diabetes Association (ADA) defines criteria for DKA resolution as glucose less than 200 mg/dL (11.1 mmol/L), and two of the following: serum bicarbonate greater than or equal to 15 mEq/L, a venous pH greater than 7.3, and a calculated anion gap less than or equal to 12 mEq/L. If the glucose reaches 200 mg/dL (11.1 mmol/L) or less, but the bicarbonate and pH are not at goal, 5% dextrose should be given to prevent hypoglycemia while the insulin infusion is continued.

Once the criteria for resolution of DKA are met, a transition to subcutaneous insulin can be undertaken. The infusion and subcutaneous insulin should overlap for a length of time appropriate to the peak of absorption of the subcutaneous insulin. For the rapid-acting insulins, the overlap should be at least 1 h. If only a long-acting insulin like glargine (Lantus®) or detemir (Levemir®) is given, the overlap should be at least 4 h.

IV Fluids

On average, patients with DKA have a total water deficit of approximately 6 L. The first step is to determine the patient's hydration status by calculation of the precise water deficit using the formula:

$$\text{water deficit (L)} = [0.6 \text{ (men) or } 0.5 \text{ (women) or } 0.45 \text{ (elderly)}]$$

$$\times \text{lean body weight (kg)} \times [(\text{plasma } [Na+] - 140)/140].$$

Normal saline is the IV fluid of choice for most adults, and a rate of 1 L/h is generally a reasonable starting point. However, a slower, more cautious approach is recommended for patients with impaired ability to manage their volume status, such as those with chronic renal insufficiency and congestive heart failure.

After 2 h of IV fluid administration, the sodium level should be evaluated. If the sodium level has not returned to normal (i.e., is still low), normal saline should be continued, and sodium reevaluated after an additional 2 h. Once the sodium level has returned to normal, the IV fluid should be changed to half-normal saline (0.45%) at a rate appropriate for continued volume repletion.

IV fluid management and electrolyte monitoring are done concomitantly with glucose and insulin management. When the blood glucose reaches 200 mg/dL (11.1 mmol/L) or less, addition of 5% dextrose to the IV fluids is warranted.

Electrolytes

Electrolytes should be monitored every 2 h during aggressive fluid and insulin administration. Once the patient is stabilized, monitoring frequency can be decreased to every 4 h. This should be continued for at least the first 24 h.

Potassium

If the potassium is low (<3.3 mEq/L), insulin should be held, and potassium chloride should be initiated intravenously (with IV fluids if desired), at 20–30 mEq/h, until potassium is more than 3.3 mEq/L.

Patients with initial potassium levels in the reference range frequently also require supplementation once insulin is begun. Although plasma potassium is maintained in the normal range, there is a total body deficit of potassium. Insulin provokes movement of potassium from the plasma into the cells, which can result in a decreased plasma potassium level once treatment is initiated.

If the initial potassium level is high, the patient's potassium should be monitored, every 2 h, without specific treatment. It is likely that the level will decrease with insulin and fluid administration.

Sodium

The initial sodium level often is low. This phenomenon does not represent true hyponatremia and will typically resolve with treatment of the hyperglycemia.

Bicarbonate

Bicarbonate administration is controversial, particularly in patients who have impaired respiratory function. However, it should be considered in patients who have severe acidosis (i.e., pH less than 6.9).

If pH is less than 6.9, dilute bicarbonate ($NaHCO_3$) with 100 mmol in 400 mL of water with 20 mEq of potassium chloride (KCl) and infuse over a period of approximately 2 h. Monitor bicarbonate every 2 h and repeat bicarbonate replacement until pH is greater than or equal to 7.0

Phosphate

Unless hypophosphatemia is severe (phosphate <1 mg/dL [< 0.32 mmol/L]) and the patient has cardiac dysfunction, anemia, or respiratory depression, phosphate is not administered. Phosphate administration in this setting can lead to severe hypocalcemia.

Key Points: DKA

- Potassium should be checked BEFORE initiation of IV insulin and frequently thereafter. Replacement should be given immediately if the level is low.
- IV regular insulin should be started promptly.
- Aggressive IV fluids are indicated as long as the patient can tolerate them; (use caution in chronic renal insufficiency and congestive heart failure).
- Monitor electrolytes: replace potassium; follow sodium and adjust IV fluids accordingly; and be judicious with bicarbonate replacement.
- Frequent glucose monitoring, with appropriate treatment adjustments.
- At least 1 h of overlap should be allowed between the first subcutaneous insulin injection and the cessation of IV insulin.
- Patients with diabetes mellitus type 1 can be in DKA even with blood glucose below 200 mg/dL (11.1 mmol/L)
- Patients with diabetes mellitus type 2 also can present with DKA, especially blacks and Hispanics/Latinos.

Hyperosmolar Hyperglycemic State

Hyperosmolar hyperglycemic state (HHS), also called hyperosmolar nonketotic hyperglycemia (HONK or HNKH), is a serious acute complication of diabetes. HHS is under diagnosed, despite its high mortality rate of approximately 11%. It is seen almost exclusively in patients with type 2 diabetes, and is more common in the elderly. The severe hyperglycemia seen in HHS results from decreased peripheral insulin effect (either from deficiency or resistance) combined with an increased counterregulatory hormone effect, and it is further compounded by volume depletion. The hyperglycemia results in glycosuria, which leads to dehydration and depletion of electrolytes.

Once a hyperglycemic emergency is diagnosed, the next step is to differentiate HHS from DKA. The major difference between the two disorders is the presence of insulin and its metabolic effects. Unlike DKA, HHS is a condition in which enough insulin is present to avoid release of fatty acids and subsequent ketoacidosis. Because of this and because HHS can present after long periods of hyperglycemia in patients with less efficient renal glucose excretion, the patients can present with very high glucose levels, sometimes greater than 1,000 mg/dL (55.5 mmol/L).

Clinical Presentation and Manifestations

The clinical presentation and manifestations of HHS include the following:

- Polyuria
- Polydipsia
- Weight loss
- Fatigue
- Slow, insidious onset of days to weeks
- Central nervous system effects, such as altered mental status or seizures
- Signs of volume depletion

  - Decreased skin turgor
  - Tachycardia
  - Hypotension
  - Low urine output

Differential Diagnosis

DKA will present with lower blood glucose. Compared with DKA, HHS usually has a blood glucose greater than 600 mg/dL (33.3 mmol/L); arterial pH usually is greater than 7.30; serum bicarbonate (NaHCO$_3$) is greater than 18 mEq/L; and ketones are usually less. Other disease entities to consider will depend on the presenting symptoms.

Precipitants

Precipitants of HHS include the following:

- New diagnosis of diabetes
- Nonadherence to medications or inadequate use of prescribed medications
- Infection
- Myocardial infarction
- Cerebroavascular accident
- Drugs
- Pancreatitis

Evaluation

Evaluation of the patient should include the following:

- Plasma glucose.
- Complete metabolic panel, with electrolytes, bicarbonate, BUN, and creatinine. Calculation of the anion gap can be helpful in distinguishing HHS from DKA; however, patients with HHS will not always have a normal anion gap. An elevated

anion gap may also be related to ingested substances, uremia, or lactic acidosis, and examination for these factors in appropriate patients, in addition to ketones, is an important component of the evaluation.

- Serum osmolality.
- Urine ketones.
- Serum ketones.
- Arterial blood gas.
- Echocardiogram, cardiac biomarkers, chest x-ray, and urine and blood cultures may be appropriate to evaluate for precipitants and sequelae, depending on the patient's presenting symptoms and comorbidities.

Laboratory Findings

Laboratory findings usually will show severe hyperglycemia and hyperosmolality, with serum osmolality greater than 320 mOsm/L. Serum bicarbonate, anion gap, and pH typically are normal, although acidosis can result from coexisting conditions, particularly if the patient is having seizures related to the hyperosmolality.

The patient may have hyponatremia, which often is artifactual. Osmotic pressure related to the high glucose level forces water into the vascular space, causing a dilutional hyponatremia, or "pseudohyponatremia." Furthermore, the high glucose can increase triglyceride levels, which can displace sodium in the plasma assay. Serum sodium level can be corrected mathematically with the following equation: Measured sodium $+(((Serum\ glucose - 100)/100) \times 1.6)$. (However, some laboratories will report the corrected sodium.) Pseudohyponatremia should correct with resolution of the hyperglycemia.

Hyperkalemia can result from lack of insulin effect at the potassium channels in the cell membranes, causing a shift of potassium to the extracellular space. (This problem is compounded in DKA because of the combined effects of inadequate insulin and acidemia.) These patients frequently have low total body potassium and will develop hypokalemia as the hyperglycemia is corrected.

Management

In brief, the following elements should be included. Detailed descriptions of each component follow.

- IV fluids
- IV insulin
- Electrolyte correction and maintenance
- Vigilance
- Treatment of precipitating factor

IV Fluids

Patients with HHS are severely dehydrated, and aggressive IV hydration is indicated. First, intravascular volume should be restored, usually with normal saline (0.9% NaCl) at 15–20 mL/kg/h, or about 1–1.5 L/h. Generally, it is necessary to maintain this rate for at least 1 h. As always, IV fluid administration requires caution in patients with impaired volume status, such as those with chronic renal insufficiency or congestive heart failure. After the first hour, the patient's volume status should be re-assessed: blood pressure, pulse rate, skin turgor, and urine output, along with evaluation of blood electrolytes and glucose.

Once the patient is hemodynamically stable and volume replete, half-normal saline (0.45% NaCl) can replace the 0.9% NaCl. The 0.45% NaCl should be continued at a reduced rate, such as 100–250 mL/h, as long as the patient remains hyperglycemic. In HHS, once the serum glucose reaches 300 mg/dL (16.6 mmol/L), 5% dextrose (D5) should be added to the 0.45% NaCl.

Insulin

IV insulin is used because of its rapid onset and facility for titration. (More discussion of titration methods is provided in Chapter 3: IV Insulin.) It is ideal to continue the insulin infusion until mental status has returned to normal, hyperosmolarity and hyperglycemia have resolved, and the patient is able to eat.

Electrolytes

Sodium

Sodium will normalize with IV fluid and insulin administration and resolution of the hyperglycemia.

Potassium

This may be elevated at presentation but will decrease with treatment with IV fluids and insulin. If initial potassium is below 3.3 mEq/L, insulin should be held and 20–30 mEq/h of potassium should be given until the potassium level is above 3.3 mEq/L. Patients with potassium levels between 3.3 and 5.2 mEq/L should receive 20–30 mEq of potassium in each liter of IV fluid. Finally, patients with potassium levels greater than 5.2 mEq/L won't need potassium supplementation initially, but the potassium level must be monitored every 2 h because of the anticipated decline in potassium with insulin therapy.

Phosphate

Phosphate can decrease with insulin treatment. As in the case of DKA, unless hypophosphatemia is severe, phosphate administration is not routinely given;

phosphate administration has been associated with development of hypocalcemia and hypomagnesemia. Although phosphate supplementation is not indicated for routine use, serum phosphate levels should be monitored to avoid cardiac, hematologic, or muscular complications.

Vigilance

Patients with HHS often require intensive monitoring and care, and an ICU setting is most appropriate. However, some institutions have intermediate care units that are equipped and have the trained personnel to manage patients with HHS. Vital signs, mental status, and hydration status should be monitored every 1–2 h while the patient is unstable and every 2–4 h for the first 24 h. Capillary glucose should be monitored hourly while the patient is on IV insulin, and electrolytes, creatinine, and serum osmolality should be checked every 2–4 h.

Key Points: HHS

- When hyperglycemic emergency is suspected, evaluation should be done immediately.
- Fluid administration is critical; volume status should be closely monitored.
- IV insulin infusion.
- Electrolyte management.
- Monitor the glucose frequently and adjust treatment as appropriate.

Bibliography

Henderson KE, Baranski TJ, Bickel PE, Clutter WE, McGill JB, eds. *The Washington Manual of Endocrinology Subspecialty Consult.* 2nd ed. Philadelphia, PA: Lippincott Williams & Wilkins; 2009.

Kitabchi AE, Umpierrez GE, Miles JM, Fisher JN. Hyperglycemic crises in adult patients with diabetes: a consensus statement from the American Diabetes Association. *Diabetes Care.* 2009;32(7):1335–1343.

Lien LF, Spratt SE, Woods Z, Osborne K, Feinglos MN. Optimizing hospital use of intravenous insulin: improved hyperglycemic management and error reduction with a new nomogram. *Endocr Pract.* 2005;11(4):240–253.

Chapter 7
Medical Nutrition Therapy in the Hospital

Sarah Gauger

Keywords Carbohydrate counting · Carbohydrate serving · Nutrition counseling

Medical nutrition therapy (MNT) is an integral component of diabetes management and of diabetes self-management education. It is usually best provided in an outpatient and home setting; however, a hospital admission provides an excellent opportunity to review, reinforce, and educate both the patient and family regarding appropriate dietary choices.

The American Diabetes Association (ADA) does not endorse any single meal plan or strict pattern of macronutrient composition. Instead, the organization recommends a dietary plan that includes carbohydrates from foods like fruits, low-fat milk, legumes, whole grains, and vegetables. Additionally, an important component of nutrition for patients with diabetes includes monitoring carbohydrates by carbohydrate counting and carbohydrate exchanges. In general, approximately 45–60 g of carbohydrates per meal can be the goal. Also, the use of low-glycemic index carbohydrates might provide moderate additional benefits. The ADA recommends that saturated fat intake should be limited to less than 7% of the total calories and that trans-fat intake should be minimized. Additionally, patients with diabetes should be encouraged to consume foods containing significant amounts of fiber, and to limit the consumption of alcohol to moderate amounts (no more than one drink/day for women and two or less for men). Finally, it is critical that any MNT be individualized and that a multidisciplinary approach is used.

Goals of MNT in the Hospital

- Support medical therapy with the aim to attain and maintain glucose control.
- Provide adequate calories throughout illness and early recovery.
- Address individual preferences based on personal, cultural, religious, and ethnic background.

S. Gauger (✉)
Duke Inpatient Diabetes Management, Duke University Medical Center, Durham, NC 27710, USA
e-mail: gauge003@mc.duke.edu

L.F. Lien et al. (eds.), *Glycemic Control in the Hospitalized Patient,*
DOI 10.1007/978-1-60761-006-9_7, © Springer Science+Business Media, LLC 2011

What Is a Carbohydrate Serving?

One "carbohydrate serving" is the same as 15 g of carbohydrate. Historically, diabetic patients counted servings as a form of carbohydrate counting, but it is now more common for patients to use grams for calculation of an insulin dose. Many hospitals still report carbohydrate servings rather than grams with their menus and food service, and some patients find this confusing. Examples of a carbohydrate serving: 4 oz fruit juice or regular soda, 1 slice of bread, 1 pint of milk, 1 small fresh fruit, such as a plum or small apple, 1/3 cup of cooked rice/pasta, 1/2 cup mashed potatoes, or 3 glucose tablets.

What Can Be Done in the Hospital?

Nutrition Consult

A nutrition consult can be invaluable for inpatient nutrition education and advice, particularly for patients who are being treated with insulin or with modified diets. However, all patients with diabetes can benefit from nutrition counseling, and this should be undertaken if it is available.

Patients taking insulin. Many of these patients, specifically those using a continuous subcutaneous insulin infusion (CSII; see Chapter 8), will need to count carbohydrates in order to determine their mealtime (bolus) insulin dosages.

Patients receiving modified diets. Patients who are receiving a "liquid diet," (in other words, a diet consisting of liquids which are often low in protein but high in carbohydrates) may experience disproportionate hyperglycemia, because simple sugars often comprise the entire calorie content of these liquids. Usually, use of a liquid diet is temporary, but some patients will need extra counseling about this issue.

Supervised Calorie Counting

Calorie counting in the hospital usually is ordered to assess for undernutrition in patients who have reasons for inadequate intake. Additional therapy can be given for patients who are not meeting their caloric needs. (Caloric need for the average hospitalized patient is 25–35 kcal/kg.) Calorie counting also can be valuable for patients who overeat. These patients often are best served by self-monitoring calorie intake with food diaries. This task also can be translated to home monitoring.

Assess for Related Comorbidities

It is important to recognize that a diabetic patient may have comorbidities that will have an impact on nutrition and nutritional goals. Some of these comorbidities include the following:

- Gastroparesis: Because of slow gastric emptying, patients should eat smaller, more frequents meals; avoid late evening snacks and high-fat foods; avoid caffeine, alcohol, and tobacco; eat slower; and eat a diet lower in fiber.
- Celiac disease (more common in association with type 1 diabetes).
- Dental disease: Will impact the dietary plan; patients with severe disease or no dentures might limit their diet to liquids and soft foods.
- Cystic fibrosis (CF)-related diabetes: Caloric restriction is never an appropriate way to control glucose in these patients. Patients with CF require nutrition in order to maintain their weight and for survival; high-fat meals usually are recommended.

Discharge Planning

Any dietary instructions given during the patient's hospital stay should be reinforced prior to discharge; this can include carbohydrate counting, food diaries, or elimination of certain high-carbohydrate products like sugar-sweetened beverages. Patients who require further education or follow-up can be referred for outpatient diabetes and nutrition counseling. Additionally, some patients do well with simple mnemonics like these:

- "Rule of Thumb"
  - Size of Thumb = 1 ounce of cheese or meat
  - Size of Fist = 1 cup of fruit or 1 medium whole raw fruit
  - Size of Fingertip = Approximately 1 teaspoon
  - Size of One Cupped Hand = 1–2 ounces of dry goods like nuts, cereal, etc.

- "Plate Method" (http://platemethod.com)
  - Fill one-half of plate with nonstarchy vegetables
  - Fill one-fourth of plate with starch source
  - Fill one-fourth of plate with protein source
  - Use fruit and milk sources for mealtime deserts

Conclusion

MNT is primarily an outpatient strategy and therefore can often end up being overlooked during a busy hospitalization. Nonetheless, it is a critical component of diabetes management, and the inpatient stay provides a unique opportunity to educate patients. MNT can be particularly useful for those patients who have little understanding of how their nutrition relates to glycemic control. Specific teaching topics for inpatient use include calorie counting and portion sizes. Finally, an inpatient nutrition consult may be requested when this resource is available.

Key Points: MNT in the Hospital

- Although the majority of MNT is directed at outpatients, it is important not to overlook the hospitalization as a teachable moment.
- Strategies for MNT in the inpatient setting include nutrition consultation and supervised calorie and carbohydrate counting.
- Discharge planning should include a review of inpatient information as well as a personalized nutrition plan for home.

Bibliography

American Diabetes Association. Diabetes nutrition recommendations for health care institutions. *Diabetes Care.* 2004;27(supp 1):S55–S57.

American Diabetes Association. Nutrition recommendations and interventions for diabetes. A position statement of the American Diabetes Association. *Diabetes Care.* 2008;31(supp 1): S61–S78.

American Diabetes Association. Standards of medical care in diabetes. *Diabetes Care.* 2009;32(supp 1):S13–S61.

Goody CM, Drago L. Using cultural competence constructs to understand food practices and provide diabetes care and education. *Diabetes Spectr.* 2009;22(1):43–47.

Idaho Plate Method. http://platemethod.com. Accessed January 19, 2010.

McKnight KA, Carter L. From trays to tube feedings: overcoming the challenges of hospital nutrition and glycemic control. *Diabetes Spectr.* 2008;21(4):233–240.

Parrish CR, Pastors JG. Nutrition FYI: nutritional management of gastroparesis in people with diabetes. *Diabetes Spectr.* 2007;20(4):231–238.

Swift CS, Boucher JL. Nutrition care for hospitalized individuals with diabetes. *Diabetes Spectr.* 2005;18(1):34–38.

Swift CS. Nutrition FYI: nutrition trends: implications for diabetes health care professionals. *Diabetes Spectr.* 2009;22(1):23–25.

Wilson DC, Kalnins D, Steward C, et al. Challenges in the dietary treatment of cystic fibrosis related diabetes mellitus. *Clin Nutr.* 2000;19(2):87–93.

Chapter 8
Insulin Pumps and Glucose Sensors in the Hospital

Sarah Gauger

Keywords Insulin pump · Continuous subcutaneous insulin infusion (CSII) · Target blood glucose range · Active insulin time · Insulin to carbohydrate ratio · Basal rate · Insulin sensitivity factor · Inpatient diabetes self-management · Bolus wizard · Continuous glucose monitoring · Glucose sensor

Understanding the Insulin Pump

An insulin pump is a small mechanical device that, through a flexible catheter, delivers insulin via a patient's subcutaneous tissue. The pump supplies a continuous infusion of insulin (continuous subcutaneous insulin infusion [CSII]). CSII is standard of care in the management of type 1 diabetes and also can be used for management of type 2 diabetes. CSII provides tremendous flexibility for patients but also requires a thorough understanding of the hardware as well as proven ability to perform diabetes self-care.

In most cases, a rapid-acting insulin, such as aspart (Novolog®), lispro (Humalog®), or glulisine (Apidra®), is used in the pump. Even though only one type of insulin is used, it functions as both the basal and bolus components. The basal insulin component is continuously infused at a programmed hourly rate, such as 0.5 units/h. (Note: Most patients will have multiple different basal rates throughout the day.) The bolus insulin component is infused at discrete times, usually with meals, and the user can direct its administration on an as-needed basis. The calculation of the insulin bolus dose is determined by a number of programmed factors:

- Target blood glucose range. Recommended ranges may differ according to the time of day (i.e., fasting, mealtime, regular exercise times); most pumps accommodate multiple target glucose ranges.

S. Gauger (✉)
Duke Inpatient Diabetes Management, Duke University Medical Center, Durham, NC 27710, USA
e-mail: gauge003@mc.duke.edu

- Active insulin time. Active insulin time is a feature that allows for the pump to factor in amounts of insulin that remain from a previous bolus. This helps to avoid "insulin stacking." The default setting usually is 5 hours, and this rarely needs to be adjusted.
- Insulin to carbohydrate ratio. This is the amount of insulin needed to cover a specific amount of carbohydrate. It is written as a ratio, with 1:15 as a representation of 1 unit per 15 g of carbohydrate.
- Insulin sensitivity factor (ISF). The ISF represents the decrease in plasma glucose that occurs with 1 unit of insulin. For example, an ISF of 50 indicates that 1 unit of insulin will decrease the glucose by 50 mg/dL (2.7 mmol/L).

The physician or provider should predetermine these factors. The bolus calculator also incorporates the current blood glucose level and the anticipated carbohydrate content of the meal, which are entered by the user at the time of the bolus.

When admitting a patient who is wearing an insulin pump, the provider should review the settings and document them in the medical record. Because understanding the pump settings is an important part of treatment and safety in the hospital, it may be necessary to consult an endocrinologist for help.

Who Can Continue CSII in the Hospital?

Patients who are eligible to continue CSII should meet the following criteria: they should be (1) fully alert with normal mental status, (2) physically able to self-manage, and (3) equipped with extra infusion sets and other necessary supplies. If there is any concern about mental status, such as fatigue or use of narcotic medications, CSII should be discontinued. Patients must have their own supplies, as even major academic hospitals do not stock supplies for insulin pumps. There are multiple types of pumps, and their use is not common enough to justify the cost of keeping supplies in the hospital.

Hospitalization is not the time for initiation of CSII, even though this question may arise during the hospital stay. Initiation of CSII requires intensive education and training that must occur over a series of outpatient appointments. Patients who are eligible and appropriate for use of CSII can be referred for outpatient consultation with a pump educator.

When Must Insulin Pumps Be Removed?

Insulin pumps should be removed during the following procedures:

- X-rays
- Computed tomography scans
- Magnetic resonance imaging scans

- Any other exposure to radiation
- Surgical procedures

The infusion set and tubing may remain in place during radiation exposure; however the pump itself must be removed.

Appropriate Documentation of Settings

There are several important pieces of data that must be obtained in order to properly care for a patient who will remain on CSII during the hospitalization. It also is important to document these data in the medical record so that all providers can be aware of the settings and other pertinent information. The following information, at a minimum, is needed to write appropriate inpatient pump self-management orders.

- Make and model of the pump
- Type of insulin
- Basal rates
- Insulin to carbohydrate ratio
- ISF
- Time and amount of the most recent bolus
- Date of the most recent infusion set change
- What is the "off-pump plan?" (Many patients using CSII will have a predetermined subcutaneous insulin regimen to be used in the case of pump failure. This regimen is a good starting point for creation of an inpatient subcutaneous insulin regimen if needed).

Example: Pump Self-Management Orders

- [Patient name] will self-administer insulin through his/her [make/model] insulin pump.
- Basal rate: At 0000 infuse [type] insulin at 1.1 units/h; then at 0300 change to 1.2 units/h; then at 0600 change to 1.1 units/h; then at 1600 change to 1.3 units/h; then at 2100 change to 0.9 units/h.
- Use the bolus wizard for bolus insulin with meals, with 1 unit of [type] insulin for every 15 g of carbohydrates.
- Use the bolus wizard to give correctional insulin, with a sensitivity factor of 50 (or give 1 unit insulin for every 50 mg/dL [2.7 mmol/L] of blood glucose over 200 mg/dL [11.1 mmol/L]).
- Change infusion set every 3 days, with first change today.
- The insulin pump, but not the infusion set, must be removed for all imaging procedures.
- Blood glucose monitoring before meals, at bedtime, and per patient request. For glucose less than 60 mg/dL (<3.3. mmol/L), treat hypoglycemia immediately, suspend the pump temporarily, and call endocrinology for assistance. For glucose

greater than 250 mg/dL (>13.8 mmol/L), also call for assistance. Record all blood glucoses and bolused insulin doses on the nurses' medication administration record.

Troubleshooting

Hyperglycemia

The following problems can occur with the infusion set:

- The tubing is not primed.
- There is air in the tubing.
- There is no insulin in the cannula.
- The infusion set is not connected to the cartridge or syringe.
- The infusion set is not connected to the patient.
- There is a leak in the infusion set.
- The cannula is dislodged or kinked.
- The infusion set has been in too long (>3 days).
- There are signs of infection (i.e., redness, discomfort, or bleeding) at the insertion site.

The following are possible problems with the pump itself:
(Many pumps have alarms that *may* provide insight when there is a problem.)

- The insulin cartridge is empty.
- The time and date on the pump are incorrect.
- The pump is not correctly programmed.
- The patient forgot to administer the most recent bolus.

The following are possible problems with the insulin:

- The insulin is expired or inactive (inactive insulin may appear cloudy or clumped).
- The insulin has been in a warm location or at room temperature for too long.
- The insulin in the cartridge is more than 3 days old.

There always is the possibility that the insulin dosage may need to be adjusted.

Hypoglycemia

Hypoglycemia should be treated promptly before causes are considered. The insulin administration via the pump should be suspended for at least 20 minutes, and 15–30 g of carbohydrates administered. Once the glucose is greater than 90 mg/dL, insulin administration may be resumed.

Insulin dose errors may occur if the bolus is too large, which may be a result of miscounted carbohydrates, inaccurate carbohydrate ratio, or other improper settings; or if the basal rate is too high.

Situational causes may include the following:

- Unanticipated fasting
- Increase in activity level, as with initiation of physical therapy or a general increase in time out of bed
- New medications
- Increased insulin absorption, which may happen in patients with improvement in edematous conditions
- Onset of menses

Prevention of Hypoglycemia

In order to prevent hypoglycemia, insulin doses, including both basal and bolus, should be reduced for patients who develop acute renal failure, hepatic failure, or other conditions that can change insulin metabolism. (A complete list can be found in Chapter 14: FAQ.) If a patient is anticipated to have rapidly changing insulin needs throughout the hospital stay, it is advisable to switch to subcutaneous insulin injections or an IV insulin infusion.

The patient's blood glucose should be monitored 6–8 times/day or more often if the patient has variable or increasing physical activity level.

Accurate carbohydrate counting is important for appropriate bolus dosing. For patients who find this difficult, a nutrition consult may be helpful.

Once a mealtime bolus is given, a corresponding carbohydrate load must be given. If a patient is inconsistent about eating meals because of nausea or any other reason, the mealtime bolus can be delivered at the end of the meal. If the patient has been given a bolus and is then unable to eat, IV dextrose should be given to prevent hypoglycemia.

Pump Site Reactions

Site Infection

Infection at the pump or sensor site is the most common complication associated with pump therapy and also is the most common reason for discontinuation of pump therapy; (in addition, please see below for more details on sensors). These infections can be rapidly progressive and must be treated immediately.

To treat, the infected infusion sets must be removed and discarded, and a new set should be placed at a site distant from the infection. Antibiotic therapy for subcutaneous infection, with consideration of resistant organisms, should be given promptly. Incision and drainage is sometimes but not always necessary; this can be determined on a case-by-case basis.

Patients with recurrent infusion site abscesses should be observed for proper insertion technique, which includes washing the area with an antibacterial soap, an antibacterial solution, or an antiseptic wipe, and letting it dry before inserting the infusion set.

Allergic Reactions

Allergic reactions may occur at infusion sites and usually are the result of adhesives or components of the infusion set needles. This most commonly occurs soon after initiation of CSII but may occur later if supply products are changed. Because pump supplies are not stocked in the hospital, no alternative supplies will be available. Thus, a patient in this situation will need subcutaneous insulin injections until he or she can see the outpatient provider to discuss options.

Transition to Subcutaneous Insulin

Conversion to subcutaneous or IV insulin often is necessary in the inpatient setting. We recommend discontinuation of CSII in the following situations:

- Patient is unable to self-manage (as determined by the patient or the provider).
- The pump malfunctions.
- A hyperglycemic emergency, such as diabetic ketoacidosis or hyperosmolar nonketotic hyperglycemia occurs.
- Patient has a critical illness.
- Patient experiences prolonged periods of fasting.
- Patient is in the perioperative period, particularly for organ transplantation.
- Total parenteral nutrition is being given to the patient.
- Glucocorticoids are being initiated.
- Patient has had a stroke.
- Patient is undergoing labor and delivery.
- Patient needs serial imaging procedures or radiation treatments.
- Other illnesses requiring prompt glucose control that are better managed with IV infusion.

The determination of route, subcutaneous versus IV, should be handled on a case-by-case basis. IV insulin infusions may be more appropriate for rapidly changing conditions or insulin needs, as well as when true insulin requirements are unclear. For more information on IV insulin, see Chapter 3: IV Insulin Infusions.

For subcutaneous insulin, the dose determination strategy is similar to that of other subcutaneous insulin regimens, which are described in Chapter 2: Subcutaneous Insulin. However, there are some differences. We describe two strategies here: the first for a patient who is eating discrete meals, the second for a patient who is fasting.

Patient Eating Discrete Meals

If the patient has an off-pump plan, this is a good place to start. If the patient does not have an off-pump plan or has changing insulin requirements, the insulin dosages can be calculated based on the patient's weight (as in Chapter 2) or estimated from the pump settings. When using the pump settings to estimate, the basal and bolus doses are calculated separately rather than as percentages of the total daily dose.

To calculate a new basal dose, it is useful to first determine the ongoing daily basal dose from the pump; most pumps report this. This basal dose can be given as one or two basal injections with long-acting insulin, like glargine (Lantus®) or detemir (Levemir®). If there have been episodes of hypoglycemia with the ongoing CSII, the basal dose should be decreased. Also, it takes several hours for long-acting insulin to reach active levels, so patients may need additional insulin before the long-acting insulin takes effect.

To calculate the mealtime dose, the carbohydrate to insulin ratio setting can be used. If the patient is in a condition to continue counting carbohydrates, the same carbohydrate ratio can be used for rapid-acting subcutaneous insulin. If the patient is unable to count carbohydrates, use the insulin to carbohydrate ratio and an estimated consistent carbohydrate content of 60 g/meal to determine the mealtime dose. For example, if the insulin to carbohydrate ratio is 1 unit/10 g carbohydrate (1:10), the patient should be given approximately 6 units of rapid-acting insulin per meal (1 unit/10 g × 60 g = 6 units). If a patient is not eating well, this dose can be reduced.

A correctional insulin scale can be created using the sensitivity factor from the pump. The ISF represents the amount of glucose reduction for each unit of insulin given. For example, a sensitivity of 50 implies that 1 unit of insulin will decrease the glucose by 50 mg/dL. A correctional insulin scale for a patient with a sensitivity factor of 50 would be in increments of 1 extra unit per 50 mg/dL greater than 150 mg/dL. Alternatively, 5% of the total daily dose of scheduled insulin can be used (as described in Chapter 2).

If a patient is getting nutrition enterally or parenterally, refer to the insulin strategy in Chapter 12: Enteral and Parenteral Nutrition.

Patient Is Fasting

Again, if the patient has an off-pump plan, this is a good place to start. Otherwise, a basal dose can be calculated by acquisition of the ongoing daily basal rate from the pump. This basal rate can be translated directly as the total basal dose into one or two doses of long-acting insulin. Alternatively, it could be divided into four doses of regular insulin, given every 6 hours. Just as for patients who are eating, if there has been hypoglycemia while on CSII and fasting, the basal dose should be reduced before administered subcutaneously.

Continuous Glucose Monitoring

Continuous glucose monitoring (CGM) is performed by a device called a glucose sensor, which is inserted and worn separately from an insulin pump. The sensor measures interstitial blood glucose levels in rapid succession to create glucose trends. It tracks glucose levels 24 hours a day, observing trends and alarming at pre-specified levels of hyper- and hypoglycemia. Typically, CGM is used by patients with diabetes who have hypoglycemia unawareness or who are pregnant, although many other patients can use it as well. The results of the Juvenile Diabetes Research Foundation trial suggest that CGM improves glycemic control without increasing hypoglycemia in patients older than age 25 years. Sensors may be worn in the arm or abdomen and, depending on the model, can remain in place for 3–7 days. CGM is not a substitute for glucose monitoring with a glucose meter; glucose meter readings are necessary for confirmation and calibration of the CGM device and should be continued multiple times daily.

Interpreting CGM Results

It is important to focus on the speed and direction of the glucose trend rather than the discrete numbers reported by the CGM. Patients with trends toward hypoglycemia and hyperglycemia can be treated accordingly.

Acknowledgment Special thanks to Jan Nicollerat, MSN, ACNS-BC, CDE, the director of Duke University's Adult Diabetes Education Program, who contributed time, resources, and wisdom during the composition of this chapter.

Bibliography

2009 Resource Guide. *Diabetes Forecast.* 62(1). http://www.forecast.diabetes.org/january-2009. Accessed January 2009.

AACE Diabetes Mellitus Clinical Practice Guidelines Task Force. American Association of Clinical Endocrinologists medical guidelines for clinical practice for the management of diabetes mellitus. *Endocr Pract.* 2007;13(suppl 1):3–68.

American Diabetes Association. Position statement: continuous subcutaneous insulin infusion. *Diabetes Care.* 2004;27(suppl 1):S110.

Animas Corporation. *My insulin pump workbook.* http://www.animascorp.com/sites/default/files/pdf/Workbook.pdf. Accessed December 3, 2009.

Burge MR, Mitchell S, Sawyer A, Schade DS. Continuous glucose monitoring: the future of diabetes management. *Diabetes Spectr.* 2008;21(2):112–119.

Farkas-Hirsch R, Levandoski LA. Implementation of continuous subcutaneous insulin infusion therapy: an overview. *Diabetes Educ.* 1988;14(5):401–406.

Lenhard MJ, Reeves GD. Continuous subcutaneous insulin infusion: a comprehensive review of insulin pump therapy. *Arch Intern Med.* 2001;161(19):2293–2300.

Medtronic MiniMed, Inc. *Getting Started Guide to CGM Training.* Northridge, CA: Medtronic Diabetes; 2007.

Parkin, C. Insulin pumps and infections. *Diabetes Forecast.* 2008;61(1). http://www.forecast.diabetes.org/magazine/ask-experts/insulin-pumps-and-infection. Accessed January 2009.

Pickup J, Keen H. Continuous subcutaneous insulin infusion at 25 years. *Diabetes Care.* 2002;25(3):593–597.

The Juvenile Diabetes Research Foundation Continuous Glucose Monitoring Study Group. Continuous glucose monitoring and intensive treatment of type 1 diabetes. *N Engl J Med.* 2008;359(14):1464–1476.

Weissber-Benchell J, Antisdel-Lomadlio J, Seshadri R. Insulin pump therapy: a meta-analysis. *Diabetes Care.* 2003;26(4):1079–1087.

Chapter 9
Non-insulin Antidiabetic Medications in the Inpatient Setting

Jennifer V. Rowell, Lekshmi T. Nair, and Mary E. Cox

Keywords Acarbose (Precose) · Bromocriptine mesylate (Cycloset®) · Exenatide (Byetta®) · Glimeperide (Amaryl®) · Glipizide (Glucotrol®) · Glyburide (Diaβeta® · Micronase®) · Liraglutide (Victoza®) · Metformin (Glucophage®) · Nateglinide (Starlix®) · Pioglitazone (Actos®) · Pramlintide (Symlin®) · Repaglinide (Prandin®) · Rosiglitazone (Avandia®) · Saxagliptin (Onglyza®) · Sitagliptin (Januvia®)

Oral and injectable non-insulin antidiabetic medications are important components of outpatient management of type 2 diabetes. They are effective and safe for plasma glucose. However, even when patients have good glycemic control at home on these medications, it is essential to evaluate their safety and utility for the management of inpatient hyperglycemia. Factors that govern glucose stability are variable for inpatients: diet and physical activity level, planned and unplanned procedures, acute/critical illness, and unexpected complications. Furthermore, antidiabetic medications typically are evaluated for efficacy in trials of outpatients who use the medications over a period of weeks or months. Most of these medications will not effectively lower glucose when used acutely in the hospital, and therefore should not be prescribed with this intent. In order to determine whether continuation of oral agents is appropriate, the provider must carefully consider the patient's anticipated length of stay and hospital course. This chapter briefly discusses the reported outpatient efficacies, including risk for hypoglycemia and other safety concerns (Tables 9.1 and 9.2).

J.V. Rowell (✉)

Division of Endocrinology, Metabolism, and Nutrition, Department of Medicine, Duke University Medical Center, Durham, NC 27710, USA

e-mail: jennifer.rowell@duke.edu

L.F. Lien et al. (eds.), *Glycemic Control in the Hospitalized Patient*,
DOI 10.1007/978-1-60761-006-9_9, © Springer Science+Business Media, LLC 2011

Table 9.1 Drug summary

Drug	A$_{1c}$ lowering (%)	Risk for hypoglycemia[a]	Common adverse effects	Contra-indications[b]	Renal dosing	Weight	Dosing	Route of administration
Metformin (Glucophage®, Glucophage XR®)	1.5–2	No	GI (nausea, vomiting, diarrhea, abdominal pain)	Abnormal CrCl, creatinine >1.5 in men, >1.4 in women. Acute or chronic metabolic acidosis	Not for use in patients with abnormal CrCl	Loss	500–1,000 mg b.i.d. XR form: 500–2,000 mg with evening meal	Oral
Pioglitazone (Actos®)	1.5	No	Edema	Symptomatic CHF	No dose adjustment necessary	Gain	15–45 mg/day	Oral
Rosiglitazone (Avandia®)	1.5	No	Edema, possible association with myocardial ischemia	Symptomatic CHF	No dose adjustment necessary	Gain	4–8 mg/day	Oral
Glipizide (Glucotrol®)	1–2	Yes	GI (nausea, vomiting, diarrhea, abdominal pain)	Type 1 diabetes, DKA	Limited data available; ↑ risk for hypoglycemia	Gain	5 mg/day to 15 mg b.i.d. (with meals)	Oral
Glyburide[c] (Diaβeta®, Micronase®)	1–2	Yes	GI (nausea, vomiting, diarrhea, abdominal pain)	Type 1 diabetes, DKA, patients treated with bosentan	Limited data available; ↑ risk for hypoglycemia	Gain	1.25–20 mg/day	Oral
Glimeperide (Amaryl®)	1–2	Yes	GI (nausea, vomiting, diarrhea, abdominal pain)	Type 1 diabetes, DKA, severe hepatic dysfunction	Limited data available; ↑ risk for hypoglycemia	Gain	1–4 mg/day	Oral

Table 9.1 (continued)

Drug	A1c lowering (%)	Risk for hypoglycemia[a]	Common adverse effects	Contra-indications[b]	Renal dosing	Weight	Dosing	Route of administration
Repaglinide (Prandin®)	0.5–1	Yes	GI (nausea, vomiting, diarrhea, abdominal pain)	Type 1 diabetes, DKA	Full dose for CrCl ≥40 mL/min, half dose for CrCl 20–40 mL/min. Not studied in patients with CrCl <20 mL/min	Gain	A1c <8% or drug naïve – 0.5–4 mg/meal A1c >8% – 1–4 mg/meal	Oral
Nateglinide (Starlix®)	0.5–1	Yes	Dizziness, elevated liver enzymes	Type 1 diabetes, DKA	No dose adjustment necessary	Gain	60–120 mg given 1–30 min before meals	Oral
Acarbose (Precose®)	0.5–1	No	GI (diarrhea, flatulence, abdominal discomfort)	Type 1 diabetes, DKA, hepatic cirrhosis, chronic intestinal diseases	Data not available; use not recommended	Neutral	25–100 mg given with the first bite of meals	Oral
Exenatide (Byetta®)	1–2	No	GI (nausea, vomiting, diarrhea, abdominal pain)	(See section on *safety* in text)	Not recommended for CrCl <30 mL/min, consider 5-mcg dose for CrCl 30–50 mL/min	Loss	5–10 mcg b.i.d., 1 h before meals	Subcutaneous
Liraglutide (Victoza®)	1–2	No	GI (nausea, vomiting, diarrhea, dyspepsia, constipation)	Personal or family history of MTC or MEN 2	No dose adjustment; limited experience in patients with abnormal renal function	Loss	0.6 mg/days for 1 week, then 1.2 mg/day[d]	Subcutaneous

Table 9.1 (continued)

Drug	A_{1c} lowering (%)	Risk for hypoglycemia[a]	Common adverse effects	Contra-indications[b]	Renal dosing	Weight	Dosing	Route of administration
Sitagliptin (Januvia®)	0.5–1	No	Rare	None except history of hypersensitivity	50 mg/day dose for CrCl 30–50 mL/min, 25 mg/days dose for CrCl <30 mL/min	Neutral	100 mg/day	Oral
Saxagliptin (Onglyza®)	0.5–1	No	Rare	None	2.5 mg/days dose for CrCl <50 mL/min	Neutral	5 mg/day	Oral
Pramlintide (Symlin®)	0.5–1	No	GI (nausea, loss of appetite), headache	Confirmed gastroparesis, hypoglycemia unawareness	No dose reduction for CrCl >20 mL/min; untested in CrCl <20 mL/min	Loss	Type 1 diabetes: 15–60 mcg t.i.d. with meals; type 2 diabetes: 60–120 mcg t.i.d. with meals	Subcutaneous
Bromocriptine mesylate (Cycloset®)	0.5	No	GI (nausea), somnolence, psychosis, orthostatic hypotension, dizziness	Syncopal migraines, lactating women	No data available	Neutral	0.8–4.8 mg/day, taken within 2 h of waking in the morning, with food	Oral

b.i.d., twice daily; CHF, congestive heart failure; CrCl, creatinine clearance; DKA, diabetic ketoacidosis; GI, gastrointestinal; MEN 2B, Multiple Endocrine Neoplasia syndrome type 2; MTC, medullary thyroid cancer; t.i.d., three times daily; XR, extended release

[a]Risk for hypoglycemia increases with addition of antidiabetic medications. Patients who are at high risk for hypoglycemia include those who are elderly, debilitated, or malnourished

[b]Each medication is contraindicated for use in patients with hypersensitivity

[c]Glynase PresTabs have different dose recommendations and are not discussed here

[d]May increase to 1.8 mg/days if not at goal on 1.2 mg/day

Table 9.2 Non-insulin antidiabetic medications and toxicities

Medication	Toxicities seen in overdose	Half-life h	Dialyzable
Metformin (Glucophage®, Glucophage XR®, Fortamet®, Riomet®, Glumetza®)[a]	Nausea, vomiting, diarrhea, pancreatitis, severe lactic acidosis, hypothermia, hypotension, tachypnea, tachycardia. Hypoglycemia is usually only seen in conjunction with other symptoms	6, XR 8–12	Yes
Piogiltazone (Actos®)	Edema, anemia, myalgia, hepatotoxicity	16–24	No
Rosiglitazone (Avandia®)	Edema, congestive heart failure, myocardial ischemia, angina, cholestatic hepatitis	3–4	No
Glipizide (Glucotrol®, Glucotrol XL®)	Hypoglycemia, nausea, diarrhea, headache, dizziness	2–4, XL 6–12	No
Glyburide (Diabeta®, Micronase®)	Hypoglycemia, nausea	10	No
Glimepiride (Amaryl®)	Hypoglycemia, nausea	5–9	No
Repaglinide (Prandin®)	Hypoglycemia, tachycardia, coma, seizures, confusion, metabolic acidosis	1	No
Nateglinide (Starlix®)	Hypoglycemia, tachycardia, coma, seizures, confusion, metabolic acidosis	1.5	Yes
Acarbose (Precose®)	Abdominal pain, diarrhea, flatulence	2	No
Exenatide (Byetta®)	Nausea, vomiting, diarrhea, anxiety, hypoglycemia; pancreatitis, renal failure	2.4	No
Liraglutide (Victoza®)	Severe nausea, vomiting	13	No
Sitagliptin (Januvia®)	Hypoglycemia, headache	12.4	Yes
Saxagliptin (Onglyza®)	No dose-related clinical adverse reactions	2.5–3.1	Yes
Pramlintide (Symlin®)	Severe nausea, vomiting, diarrhea, vasodilation, dizziness	0.8	No
Bromocriptine mesylate (Cycloset®)	Nausea, vomiting, constipation, diaphoresis, dizziness, pallor, severe hypotension, malaise, confusion, lethargy, drowsiness, delusions, hallucinations, and repetitive yawning	6	No

XR, extended release

[a]Fortamet® and Glumetza® are extended-release preparations

Biguanides

Metformin (Glucophage®, Glucophage XR®)

Mechanism and Efficacy

Metformin improves glucose tolerance by decreasing hepatic glucose production, decreasing intestinal absorption of glucose, and increasing peripheral glucose uptake and utilization. The clinical efficacy of metformin is dependent on the amount of insulin resistance that is present; a typical reduction in A_{1C} is about 1.5–1.8%.

Safety

For outpatients, the major adverse effect of metformin is its propensity to cause gastrointestinal (GI) symptoms, particularly diarrhea. However, for inpatients, the major concern is the risk for lactic acidosis. Compared with a previous biguanide phenformin, which is no longer on the market, the incidence of lactic acidosis with metformin is rare. However, it is life threatening, and, thus, use of metformin should be avoided in patients at risk. These include the following:

- Renal failure, acute or chronic: Creatinine level greater than 1.5 mg/dL in men or 1.4 mg/dL in women, or abnormal creatinine clearance. Because aging is associated with reduced renal function, absolute creatinine levels may not be reflective of abnormal creatinine clearance in elderly patients
- Liver dysfunction
- Acute or chronic metabolic acidosis
- Cardiac disease, including congestive heart failure (CHF; acute or chronic under drug treatment), myocardial infarction, cardiovascular collapse
- History of alcohol abuse
- Severe infection
- Hypoxia from any cause

Metformin does not increase risk for hypoglycemia when used alone, although it may increase the risk for hypoglycemia when combined with other antidiabetic medications, including insulin. Elderly, debilitated, and malnourished patients are particularly susceptible to hypoglycemia.

Inpatient Considerations

Most providers choose to discontinue metformin during hospitalization because of the safety issues above. If metformin is continued, its use should be avoided at least 48 h before and after imaging procedures with iodinated contrast or surgical procedures. The same is true for concomitant use of medications that are known to affect renal function. Metformin may be restarted once renal function has been reevaluated and found to be normal.

Thiazolidinediones

Pioglitazone (Actos®), Rosiglitazone (Avandia®)

Mechanism and Efficacy

Thiazolidinedione (TZD) medications share a common mechanism, which is to decrease peripheral insulin resistance in muscle and adipose tissues as well as inhibit hepatic gluconeogenesis. Specifically, these compounds are agonists for peroxisome proliferator–activated-receptor-γ (PPARγ), which modulates transcription of a number of insulin-responsive genes.

As with metformin, the efficacy of TZD therapy differs depending on an individual patient's insulin resistance. However, a typical A_{1C} reduction is approximately 1.5%.

Safety

The most common adverse effect of the TZD class is an increase in fluid retention, which can worsen peripheral edema and CHF. Patients with symptomatic CHF should not use TZDs.

The first member of the TZD class, troglitazone, was withdrawn from the market because of rare but serious hepatotoxicity. The newer agents, pioglitazone and rosiglitazone, do not appear to share this adverse effect. However, hepatic monitoring is recommended for patients at initiation of these medications, and periodically thereafter, as rare patients have been noted to have hepatic enzyme elevations greater than three times the upper limit of normal.

TZDs have not been found to cause hypoglycemia when used independently but may be associated with hypoglycemia when combined with other agents like insulin or sulfonylureas.

In a meta-analysis of 42 clinical studies, rosiglitazone, as compared with placebo, was found to be associated with an increased risk for myocardial ischemic events (Nissen and Wolski, 2007). To date, further study has not confirmed or excluded this risk. Available data on pioglitazone has not confirmed a similar risk. Rosiglitazone should be used with caution in patients who have high risk for coronary artery disease.

Inpatient Considerations

TZD's generally are safe for continuation during hospitalization, as long as the patient continues with a regular diet, and none of the safety concerns listed above apply. It should be noted that TZDs are ineffective for acute management of hyperglycemia because the time to steady state is about 6 weeks.

Sulfonylureas

Glipizide (Glucotrol®), Glimepiride (Amaryl®), Glyburide (Diaβeta®, Glynase PresTabs®, Micronase®)

Mechanism and Efficacy

The sulfonylureas are the traditional insulin secretagogues. They work by influencing closure of an adenosine triphosphate (ATP)-dependent potassium channel on the β(beta)-cell membrane. This channel closure results in a series of effects that culminate in insulin release. Notably, release of insulin in response to sulfonylurea administration is not related to blood glucose level. Treatment with a sulfonylurea drug can be expected to lower the A_{1C} by 1–2%.

Safety

The most common adverse reaction to sulfonylurea drugs is GI disturbance, such as nausea and diarrhea or constipation. The most common serious reaction with these medications is hypoglycemia; all sulfonylurea drugs are capable of producing severe hypoglycemia. (Table 9.3).

Table 9.3 Risk factors for hypoglycemia

Adrenal or pituitary insufficiency
Advanced age
Alcohol ingestion
Hepatic insufficiency
Malnourishment or low calorie intake
Multiple glucose-lowering drugs
Renal insufficiency
Severe or prolonged exercise

The package insert for sulfonylurea drugs contains a warning regarding the results of the University Group Diabetes Program (Diabetes, 1970), that administration of sulfonylureas is associated with increased cardiovascular mortality, as compared with treatment with diet alone or diet plus insulin. This association remains controversial.

Inpatient Considerations

The most important inpatient consideration with sulfonylureas is the potential for hypoglycemia, particularly in patients with acute or chronic renal dysfunction. Because hospitalized patients are at particular risk for hypoglycemia, sulfonylureas must be used with caution.

Meglitinides

Repaglinide (Prandin®), Nateglinide (Starlix®)

Mechanism and Efficacy

Although the meglitinides are chemically unrelated to the traditional insulin secretagogues, their mechanism of action is similar. The meglitinides also function to close the ATP-dependent potassium channels in the β-cell membrane, resulting in a number of events that culminate in insulin secretion. A typical A_{1C} reduction for a meglitinide medication is approximately 0.5–1%.

Safety

As with the sulfonylureas, meglitinide-induced insulin secretion is not related to plasma glucose levels, and hypoglycemia can result from its administration. Its use should be avoided in patients who are not eating or who are at risk for hypoglycemia

(Table 9.3). Other adverse effects of meglitinides are similar to those of sulfony-lureas, and are primarily gastrointestinal. Repaglinide appears to be safe if slowly up-titrated in patients with impaired hepatic function, but nateglinide has not been studied in this population.

Inpatient Considerations

The most important inpatient consideration for meglitinides is the potential for hypoglycemia. For this reason, as with the sulfonylureas, the meglitinides should be used with caution in hospitalized patients.

α (alpha)-Glucosidase Inhibitor

Acarbose (Precose®)

Mechanism and Efficacy

The anti-hyperglycemic effect of acarbose results from inhibition of disaccharide cleavage in the small intestine, which delays carbohydrate absorption. This effect results in a decrease in postprandial hyperglycemia. A typical A_C reduction with acarbose is 0.5–1%. It is important to note that the mechanism of acarbose is uniquely effective for patients who are eating and will not lower glucose levels in patients who are fasting. Its efficacy is also related to the amount of carbohydrate in the diet.

Safety

The most common adverse effects with acarbose are gastrointestinal: diarrhea, flatulence, and abdominal discomfort. These may decrease in severity over weeks of treatment. However, because of these actions, this drug is contraindicated in patients with chronic intestinal diseases. Also, there have been reports of patients with elevated transaminases while taking acarbose, and its use is not recommended in patients with cirrhosis. Acarbose does not cause hypoglycemia as mono-therapy. Because acarbose inhibits disaccharide cleavage, orally administered disaccharides such as sucrose can not be used to treat hypoglycemia when acarbose has been administered. Orally administered glucose tablets or glucose gel, as well as other non-oral methods of hypoglycemia treatment, should be effective.

Inpatient Considerations

As above, acarbose is uniquely effective in patients who are eating regular meals with significant portions of carbohydrate. For this reason, it is infrequently used in the inpatient setting, given the propensity for missed meals.

Glucagon-Like Peptide-1 Analogs

Exenatide (Byetta®), Liraglutide (Victoza®)

Mechanism and Efficacy

Exenatide and liraglutide exert their actions by mimicking endogenous glucagon-like peptide (GLP)-1; in fact, liraglutide shares 97% homology with human GLP-1. The effects of GLP-1 receptor agonism are to increase glucose-dependent pancreatic insulin secretion, suppress glucagon secretion, decrease the rate of gastric emptying, and induce central appetite suppression. These effects are dependent on the plasma glucose level and will not occur if glucose levels are below 65 mg/dL. Exenatide is typically effective for lowering A_{1C} by 1–2%, and liraglutide has shown similar efficacy.

Safety

GI adverse effects are common, primarily with nausea and vomiting. GI effects may be more pronounced in patients with diabetic gastroparesis. In such patients, caution should be used. Because of the glucose-dependent mechanism, hypoglycemia does not occur when exenatide is used as mono-therapy.

Based on postmarketing data, exenatide has been associated with episodes of pancreatitis. In preclinical trials, liraglutide was also associated with a slightly increased risk of pancreatitis over placebo. Although this risk has not been confirmed to be greater than that with other antidiabetic medications on subsequent retrospective analysis, it currently is recommended that the GLP-1 analogs be avoided in patients with a history of pancreatitis, and that the drugs be discontinued immediately in patients who develop signs or symptoms of pancreatitis while using exenatide or liraglutide.

Liraglutide causes development of medullary thyroid carcinoma at clinically relevant exposures in rat and mouse models. It has not conclusively been found to have this effect on humans; however, it is prudent to avoid its use in patients with family or personal history of medullary thyroid carcinoma or multiple endocrine neoplasia syndrome type 2B.

Inpatient Considerations

Neither of these medications causes hypoglycemia when used as mono-therapy. Exenatide is given in relation to meals, and this is likely to be a problem in the inpatient setting. Liraglutide is not given in relation to meals and may be easier to administer in the hospital. However, there are no data as to whether one may be substituted for the other. Because of the effects on gastric emptying, use of GLP-1 analogs may interfere with absorption of oral contraceptive pills and antibiotics; they should be given 2 h before or after administration of exenatide or liraglutide. In general, there is only limited experience with the use of these agents in the inpatient setting.

Dipeptidyl Peptidase-4 Inhibitors

Sitagliptin (Januvia®), Saxagliptin (Onglyza®)

Mechanism and Efficacy

Dipeptidyl peptidase (DPP)-4 inhibitors increase GLP-1 levels by inhibiting the enzyme responsible for endogenous GLP-1 metabolism. The increase in endogenous GLP-1 results in an increase in glucose-dependent pancreatic insulin secretion. However, other effects of GLP-1 analogs, such as satiety, are not as evident with the DPP-4 inhibitor medications. Anticipated improvements in A_{1C} are in the order of 0.5–1%.

Safety

The DPP-4 inhibitors are relatively free from common adverse effects. Because of the glucose-dependent mechanism of action, risk for hypoglycemia is low. As for GLP-1 agonists, there have been postmarketing reports that associate use of DPP-4 inhibitors with episodes of pancreatitis. Follow-up retrospective data has not confirmed this association, but it is still reasonable to avoid these medications for patients who have a history of pancreatitis. Finally, a history of hypersensitivity is a contraindication for these agents.

Inpatient Considerations

The DPP-4 inhibitors have few side effects, do not cause hypoglycemia, and do not need to be administered in relation to meals. However, it should be noted that they may not effectively treat acute hyperglycemia, which still is best addressed with use of insulin.

Amylin Analog

Pramlintide (Symlin®)

Mechanism and Efficacy

Pramlintide exerts its action by mimicking the physiologic effects of amylin (i.e., to suppress postprandial glucagon secretion, delay gastric emptying, and influence satiety via effects on the central nervous system). These combined effects result in a reduced postprandial glucose excursion. Pramlintide can be expected to lower the A_{1C} by 0.5–1%. Pramlintide is unique among the non-insulin antidiabetic agents because it also has been found to be effective in patients with type 1 diabetes.

Safety

Pramlintide's most common adverse effects are nausea, loss of appetite, and headache. When used alone, it does not increase risk for hypoglycemia. It should be noted that, although pramlintide and prandial insulin can be administered at the same time, they should not be given in the same syringe.

Inpatient Considerations

Pramlintide may be continued along with prandial insulin for patients who are eating meals in the hospital. However, it should be held whenever meals are held. Like the other non-insulin antidiabetic drugs, it is unlikely to be as effective as insulin at treatment of acute hyperglycemia.

Dopamine Agonist

Bromocriptine Mesylate (Cycloset®)

Mechanism and Efficacy

Bromocriptine mesylate is a dopamine agonist that is indicated for treatment of prolactinoma and Parkinson's disease. It recently achieved an FDA indication for treatment of type 2 diabetes as well. The mechanism of glucose lowering is not well understood but is thought to be a central signaling phenomenon. It can be expected to lower A_{1C} by approximately 0.5%.

Safety

GI side effects, primarily nausea, are common with bromocriptine. At higher doses than those prescribed for diabetes therapy, central effects have been noted, including somnolence, orthostatic hypotension, dizziness, and psychosis. It is not recommended to use bromocriptine for patients with low blood pressure or psychotic disorders. Furthermore, fibrotic complications, such as retroperitoneal fibrosis and pulmonary fibrosis, have been noted with other formulations of bromocriptine. Risk for hypoglycemia with bromocriptine is low.

Inpatient Considerations

Because bromocriptine's mechanism of action on lowering glucose is not well understood, and because there is little experience with it for this indication, it is not recommended to use bromocriptine in hospitalized patients.

Non-insulin Antidiabetic Medications and Cardiovascular Health

Historically, the antidiabetic medications had been presumed to improve cardiovascular health by way of improving glycemic control. However, in recent years, this has come into question, and the FDA has required that prescribing information for these drugs explicitly state whether the drug has been associated with improved cardiovascular outcomes. Data on specific drugs remain controversial, and more research needs to be done in this area. For now, these drugs should not be prescribed for the explicit purpose of cardiovascular protection.

Key Points

- Non-insulin antidiabetic agents are quite useful for outpatient management, but have limited use in the inpatient setting for reasons described here.
- Acute intervention with insulin is the safest and most rapid means for achieving glycemic control in the hospital.

Bibliography

Actos [Prescribing Information]. Deerfield, IL: Takeda Pharmaceuticals America, Inc.; 2008.

Ahmad SR, Swann J. Exenatide and rare adverse events: letter to the editor. *N Engl J Med.* 2008;358(18):1970–1971.

Amaryl [package insert]. Bridgewater, NJ: Sanofi-aventis; 2009.

Avandia [prescribing information]. Research Triangle Park, NC: GlaxoSmithKline; 2008.

Byetta [prescribing information]. San Diege, CA: Amylin Pharmaceuticals; 2009.

Cycloset [prescribing information]. Tiverton, RI: VeroScience, LLP; 2009.

Diaβeta [package insert]. Bridgewater, NJ: Sanofi-aventis US, LLC; 2009.

Donner TW, Flammer KM. Diabetes management in the hospital. *Med Clin North Am.* 2008;92(2):407–425, ix–x.

Drucker DJ. The incretin system: glucagon-like peptide-1 receptor agonist and dipeptidyl peptidase-4 inhibitors in type 2 diabetes. *Lancet.* 2006;368:1696–1702.

Edelman SV, Caballero L. Amylin replacement therapy in patients with type I diabetes. *Diabetes Educ.* 2006;32(3):119S–127S.

Edelman SV, Darsow T, Frias JP. Pramlintide in the treatment of diabetes. *J Clin Pract.* 2006;60(12):1647–1653.

Gallwitz B. Exenatide in type 2 diabetes: treatment effects in clinical studies and animal study data. *J Clin Pract.* 2006;60(12):1654–1661.

Glucophage and Glucophage XR [package insert]. Princeton, NJ: Bristol-Myers Squibb Company; 2006.

Glucotrol [package insert]. New York, NY: Pfizer; 2009.

Glumetza [package insert]. Menlo Park, CA: Depomed, Inc; 2006.

Januvia [prescribing information]. White House Station, NJ: Merck, 2006.

Kruger DF, Martin CL, Sadler CE. New insights into glucose regulation. *Diabetes Educ.* 2006;32(2):221–228.

Lien LF, Bethel MA, Feinglos MN. In-hospital management of type 2 diabetes mellitus. *Med Clin North Am.* 2004;88(4):1085–1105, xii.

Martin C. The physiology of amylin and insulin: maintaining the balance between glucose secretion and glucose uptake. *Diabetes Educ.* 2006;32(3):101S–104S.

McMahon GT. State-of-the-art diabetes care: where we've been, where we are, and where we're going. *Adv Stud Med.* 2005;5:S912–S918.

Mikhail NE. Is exenatide a useful addition to diabetes therapy? *Endocr Prac.* 2006;12(3):307–314.

Nissen SE, Wolski K. Effect of rosiglitazone on the risk of myocardial infarction and death from cardiovascular causes. N Engl J Med. 2007;356(24):2457–2471.

Odegard PS, Setter SM, Iltz JL. Update in the pharmacologic treatment of diabetes mellitus: focus on pramlintide and exenatide. *Diabetes Educ.* 2006;32(5):693–712.

Onglyza [package insert]. Princeton, NJ: Bristol-Myers Squibb Company; 2009.

Owen SK. Amylin replacement therapy in patients with insulin-requiring type 2 diabetes. *Diabetes Educ*. 2006;32(3):105S–110S.

Prandin [package insert]. Princeton, NJ: Novo Nordisk; 2006.

Precose [prescribing information]. Wayne, NJ: Bayer HealthCare Pharmaceuticals; 2008.

Saudek CD. Assessing new options for the treatment of diabetes: a review for practicing clinicians. *Adv Stud Med*. 2005;5:S910–S911.

Starlix [prescribing information]. Stein, Switzerland: Novartis Pharma Stein AG; 2008.

Symlin [prescribing information]. San Diego, CA: Amylin Pharmaceuticals; 2008.

Umpierrez GE, Palacio A, Smiley D. Sliding scale insulin use: myth or insanity? *Am J Med*. 2007;120(7):563–567.

Victoza [prescribing information]. Bagsvaerd, Denmark: Novo Nordisk A/S, 2010.

Chapter 10
Hypoglycemia

Melanie E. Mabrey, Mary E. Cox, and Lillian F. Lien

Keywords Hypoglycemia · Glucagon · Gluconeogenesis · Neuroglycopenic · Whipple's triad · Counterregulatory hormones · Hypoglycemia unawareness · 50% dextrose (D50) · Glucose monitoring

Hypoglycemia is the primary limiting factor for achieving optimal glucose control for patients both in and out of the hospital. Certainly, concerns about hypoglycemia are warranted given the acute danger of hypoglycemia as well as the potential for long-term sequelae. Although diabetes may be only one of many comorbidities for patients admitted to the hospital, practical measures can be taken that will prompt recognition and treatment if hypoglycemia occurs. This chapter addresses three components of inpatient diabetes management with respect to hypoglycemia: recognition, treatment, and prevention.

Recognition of Hypoglycemia

Because the human body preferentially uses glucose as fuel, there are several complementary protective mechanisms in response to low circulating blood glucose levels. In the early phase of hypoglycemia, pancreatic alpha cells respond by releasing glucagon. Glucagon stimulates hepatocytes to break down stored glycogen, releasing glucose, while also activating hepatic gluconeogenesis. These mechanisms often suffice to raise blood glucose to normal levels, although glucagon response may decline with longstanding disease, particularly in patients with type 1 diabetes. In prolonged hypoglycemia, as in patients who have taken a disproportionate amount of insulin, or for those who are malnourished and have low hepatic glucose stores, other counterregulatory mechanisms are triggered: release of epinephrine, norepinephrine, growth hormone, and cortisol. These counterregulatory hormones

M.E. Mabrey (✉)
Duke Inpatient Diabetes Management, Department of Advanced Clinical Practice, Duke University Hospital, Durham, NC, USA; Duke University Schools of Nursing and Medicine, Duke University Medical Center, Durham, NC, USA
e-mail: mabre002@mc.duke.edu

L.F. Lien et al. (eds.), *Glycemic Control in the Hospitalized Patient*,
DOI 10.1007/978-1-60761-006-9_10, © Springer Science+Business Media, LLC 2011

can raise blood glucose and also result in detectable symptoms and signs, termed *neurogenic* or autonomic symptoms of hypoglycemia. Other symptoms, due directly to the brain's deprivation of glucose, are termed *neuroglycopenic*.

The diagnosis of true hypoglycemia only can be confirmed in patients for whom the three components of Whipple's triad are observed: (1) signs or symptoms of hypoglycemia, (2) low blood glucose level, and (3) resolution of signs and symptoms with normalization of the blood glucose level. However, it is important to recognize that symptoms of hypoglycemia vary from patient to patient. Some patients will have a complete absence of symptoms, termed *hypoglycemia unawareness*; this is not rare and has many possible causes (Table 10.1). Some patients present with typical neurogenic/autonomic symptoms, which may include tremor, diaphoresis, nervousness or anxiety, and palpitations. Others may experience neuroglycopenic symptoms such as dizziness, sleepiness, weakness, and confusion. Some patients will experience hunger or a change in vision. Yet others will demonstrate extreme changes in behavior which may vary from inappropriate laughter, to belligerence or violence, to complete loss of consciousness or seizure.

Table 10.1 Causes of hypoglycemia unawareness

- Recent history of frequent hypoglycemia
- Rapid decline in blood glucose
- Alcohol consumption
- Use of medications like β (beta) -blockers, which may blunt symptoms
- Long duration of diabetes
- Significant stress or depression

When a patient exhibits signs or symptoms that are suspected to be related to hypoglycemia, the blood glucose level must be checked immediately. Point-of-care glucose testing is usually employed so that appropriate treatment can ensue promptly. Hypoglycemia must be considered for any patient who is treated with insulin or other anti-hyperglycemic medication; in the hospital, "insulin reactions" are the cause of almost all hypoglycemic events. Hypoglycemia is defined in patients treated with these medications as a blood glucose level of less than 70 mg/dL. (Some nondiabetic patients, particularly young women, can have normal blood glucose levels much lower than 70 mg/dL after periods of fasting. These patients are typically asymptomatic.) Once hypoglycemia is identified, treatment should begin immediately (Table 10.2).

Treatment of Hypoglycemia

The treatment for all hypoglycemic events is administration of glucose. The route and amount of administration will depend on the glucose level as well as the patient's level of consciousness and available access (Table 10.2 and Fig. 10.1). Consider the "rule of 15s:" 15 g of carbohydrate will raise the glucose about 15 mg/dL in about 15 min. Obviously the "rule of 15s" is just a starting point, and frequent monitoring is required until the blood glucose is observed to return to normal.

Table 10.2 Steps to confirm and treat hypoglycemia

1	Repeat the glucose measurement right away to confirm—repeat point-of-care testing glucose can be done quickly, and plasma glucose can be sent for confirmation if desired
2	Determine the patient's access route
3	When treating a patient for whom oral intake is safe, administer 15 g of carbohydrate orally
4	If hypoglycemic coma or seizure occur, immediately administer one ampule of 50% dextrose (D50) intravenously and continue close patient monitoring
5	After treatment, glucose measurement should be repeated in 15–20 min. If the blood glucose is still less than 70 mg/dL (3.8 mmol/L), re-treat. Repeat the process until glucose is greater than 70 mg/dL (3.8 mmol/L)
6	If the glucose remains less than 70 mg/dL (3.8 mmol/L) after three treatments, consider a continuous 5 or 10% dextrose IV infusion
7	Determine the cause of the hypoglycemic episode and whether insulin or other medications need to be adjusted
8	Continue subsequent glucose monitoring to ensure that the patient does not have rebound hyperglycemia after the occurrence or treatment of hypoglycaemia

Source: Duke University Hospital Glycemic Safety Committee, courtesy of Mary Jane Stillwagon, BSN, RN

Patients who are able to take glucose by mouth should consume 15 g of simple carbohydrates, often in the form of three to four glucose tablets, a tube of glucose gel, or 4 ounces of juice or regular soda. Patients with profoundly low blood glucose (i.e., <40 mg/dL) may require at least 30 or 45 g of carbohydrates for normalization. For patients who are unable to take oral glucose but who have an IV in place, concentrated IV 50% dextrose (D50) is the preferred treatment. D50 comes in ampules of 50 mL, or 25 g dextrose. A starting point for D50 dosing is to give a half ampule, or 25 mL (12.5 g), of D50 by IV push, to treat hypoglycemia in the range of 41–69 mg/dL. A whole ampule is given for blood glucose less than 40 mg/dL. D50 also can be given through a feeding tube when mixed with equal parts of water.

If it is not feasible to give glucose by mouth, and the patient does not have a feeding tube or an IV, 1 mg of glucagon given by intramuscular injection is the necessary treatment. Glucagon may cause vomiting, so it is a choice of last resort, and appropriate precautions should be taken to prevent aspiration if the patient is unconscious. Glucagon may not be effective in patients who are malnourished and have low hepatic glycogen stores, so a route of access for D50 should be pursued promptly.

Once glucose (dextrose) has been given, the patient's glucose should be monitored until the level is observed to be above 70 mg/dL. If the episode of hypoglycemia occurs between meals, an additional form of glucose along with protein should be given (i.e., peanut butter and crackers, milk, half a sandwich, or cheese and crackers). If the hypoglycemia is observed just before mealtime, the regular meal and mealtime insulin can be given once the blood glucose has stabilized. Once an episode of hypoglycemia has been observed and treated, appropriate steps should be taken to determine the etiology and direct future prevention.

It is worth noting that the patient may continue to experience mild symptoms even after the blood glucose level has risen. Reassurance can be helpful, concurrent with close monitoring. Certainly, resolution of symptoms will make the patient more

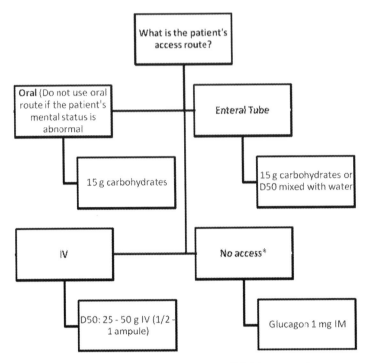

Abbreviations: D50, 50% dextrose; IV, intravenous; IM, intramuscular.

*If a patient does not have access, this should be discussed promptly with the care team. Source: Duke University Hospital Glycemic Safety Committee, courtesy of Mary Jane Stillwagon, BSN, RN.

Fig. 10.1 Hypoglycemia algorithm. Decision about therapy should be based on the patient's mental status and access routes, using the least invasive method available. Abbreviations: D50, 50% dextrose; IV, intravenous; IM, intramuscular. *If a patient does not have access, this should be discussed promptly with the care team. Source: Duke University Hospital Glycemic Safety Committee, courtesy of Mary Jane Stillwagon, BSN, RN

comfortable, but it also is important to avoid giving carbohydrates in an amount that greatly exceeds that required to normalize glucose. Extra food items, together with the counterregulatory hormone response, can lead to severe rebound hyperglycemia.

Prevention of Hypoglycemia

Prevention of hypoglycemia in the hospital must be a priority, while keeping in balance the need for appropriate blood glucose control. There are three components of hypoglycemia prevention: (1) appropriate insulin or medication dosages, adjusted for conditions that increase risk for hypoglycemia; (2) appropriate blood glucose targets; and (3) appropriate blood glucose monitoring frequency.

Appropriate Insulin or Medication Dosages

A strategy for choosing a starting dose schedule for insulin is detailed in Chapter 2: Subcutaneous Insulin. To avoid hypoglycemia, it is important to reevaluate the dosing schedule at least once a day. There are two common scenarios for which insulin doses should be decreased: episodes of hypoglycemia and change in nutrition status or temporary fasting (i.e., nothing by mouth [NPO] status).

Any Episode of Hypoglycemia

With episodes of hypoglycemia, insulin reduction often is appropriate, but complete discontinuation is rarely indicated, even with the immediately subsequent dose. Counterregulatory hormones as well as hypoglycemia treatments often cause hyperglycemia.

Change in Nutrition Status, or Temporary Fasting (i.e., NPO Status)

In the hospital, NPO status is implemented most commonly prior to procedures or operations. Generally, oral anti-hyperglycemic medications are held only on the morning of the procedure and can be restarted once eating resumes. Metformin, however, should be held at least 48 h prior to scheduled procedures, and it should be held for at least 48 h after. (Further information on non-insulin medications can be found in Chapter 9: Alternatives to Insulin.) Periprocedural insulin management should incorporate continuation of basal insulin and a pause in prandial insulin, as shown in Table 10.3.

Patients receiving enteral or parenteral nutrition may have unexpected interruptions in feeding. When interruptions occur after full-dose scheduled insulin has been given, the risk for hypoglycemia is high. To prevent hypoglycemia in this setting, Duke Hospital now uses the algorithm given in Fig. 10.2.

Other reasons to decrease insulin might include the following:

- Downward blood glucose trend
- Acute renal failure
- Acute hepatic failure
- Severe sepsis or shock
- Increased physical activity
- Taper of steroid dosage
- Improvement in infectious illness

Appropriate Glucose Targets

The diabetes field is rich with discussion regarding optimal glycemic targets. The challenge in the inpatient setting is to prevent hyperglycemia and its known complications (postoperative infection rate increase, morbidity, and mortality), while also avoiding hypoglycemia and its associated risks. Although the issue requires further

Table 10.3 Insulin adjustments to prevent hypoglycemia when a patient is not eating prior to a procedure or operation

Type of insulin	Action: night before procedure	Action: morning of procedure
Regular insulin • Humulin R®, Novolin R® • ReliOn R®	Give full dose with evening meal or as scheduled. If the evening meal is not given, give half dose at the scheduled time	Give half dose at the scheduled time
NPH insulin • Humulin N®, Novolin N® • ReliOn N®	Give full dose at bedtime	If a patient has scheduled AM NPH insulin, give half dose at the scheduled time
Premixed insulin • Humulin® 70/30™ • Novolin® 70/30™ • Humalog® 75/25™ • Novolog® 70/30™	Give full dose with evening meal or as scheduled. If the evening meal is not given, give half dose at the scheduled time	Give half dose at the scheduled time
Rapid-acting insulin • Aspart (Novolog®) • Glulisine (Apidra®) • Lispro (Humalog®)	Give full dose with evening meal. If the evening meal is not given, do not give the insulin	Do not give
Long-acting insulin • Glargine (Lantus®) • Detemir (Levemir®)	If the regimen includes long-acting insulin and rapid-acting insulin, give full dose at bedtime or as scheduled If the regimen includes long-acting insulin and oral medications or long-acting insulin alone, give half dose	Same as the night before
Continuous subcutaneous insulin infusion (CSII)	Continue current settings	Consult patient's diabetes care provider

research, it is reasonable to pursue pre-meal blood glucose less than 140 mg/dL (7.8 mmol/L), in conjunction with random blood glucose of less than 180 mg/dL (10.0 mmol/L) as straightforward goals that can apply to most inpatients.

These glucose target ranges are appropriate for "most" patients, but the choice of glucose target range requires clinical judgment as well. For example, patients with low risk for hypoglycemia, such as those taking only metformin, may have a target range of 80–120 mg/dL. Conversely, those of advanced age or with hypoglycemia unawareness may have goal glucose levels closer to 200 mg/dL. It is appropriate to make this determination for each individual patient and document the target range in the patient's record so that all providers are working toward the same end.

Appropriate Glucose Monitoring Frequency

The frequency of monitoring is usually determined by the insulin-dosing schedule, with a minimum of four point-of-care glucose tests in 24 h. Typically, blood

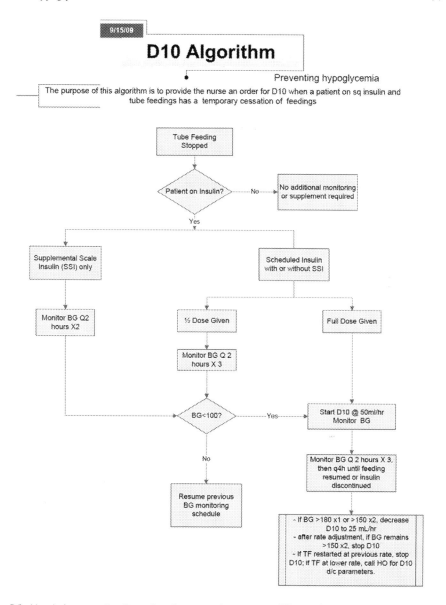

BG, blood glucose; d/c, discontinuation; sq, subcutaneous; TF, tube feeding; HO, house officer.

Source: Duke University Hospital Glycemic Safety Committee, courtesy of Mary Jane Stillwagon, BSN, RN.

Fig. 10.2 Algorithm for administration of dextrose 10% (D10) while a patient's enteral feeding is held. Abbreviations: BG, blood glucose; d/c, discontinuation; sq, subcutaneous; TF, tube feeding; HO, house officer. Source: Duke University Hospital Glycemic Safety Committee, courtesy of Mary Jane Stillwagon, BSN, RN

glucose monitoring takes place just prior to insulin administration, so that appropriate correctional insulin also may be given. Additional overnight monitoring, at around 3 AM, can be useful to determine whether undetected hypoglycemia is occurring overnight. Monitoring may be required more frequently in patients whose insulin requirements are changing, who are pregnant, or in patients to whom insulin has been given and feeding is unexpectedly interrupted. Furthermore, monitoring should occur immediately any time hypoglycemia is suspected.

Some patients have increased risk for development of hypoglycemia. Risk factors include the following:

- High doses of insulin
- Hypoglycemia unawareness
- Renal failure
- History of erratic blood glucose
- History of pancreatic disorders
- Advanced age
- Hepatic failure
- Heart failure
- Change in nutritional status, such as temporary NPO or change in rate or pattern of enteral or parenteral nutrition
- Adrenal insufficiency, chronic glucocorticoid use, or glucocorticoids in tapering dosages
- Severe sepsis, shock, or multiorgan failure
- Malignancy or catabolic state
- Malabsorption
- Improvement in states of physiologic stress and resultant decrease in insulin resistance
- Increased physical activity
- Thyroid dysfunction

Key Points: Hypoglycemia

- The official diagnosis of hypoglycemia is the presence of Whipple's Triad.
- In the hospital, a practical cut-off for hypoglycemia is blood glucose less than 70 mg/dL.
- Symptoms of hypoglycemia vary, so it is important to have a high index of suspicion and monitor glucose with any unusual symptoms or behavior.
- For hypoglycemia treatment, remember the "rule of 15s": 15 g of glucose will raise the blood glucose about 15 mg/dL in about 15 min.
- Treatment options in order of preference are (1) oral glucose (15 g), (2) D50 by IV or feeding tube, and (3) intramuscular glucagon (last resort).

- An ounce of prevention is worth a pound of cure. Insulin regimens must be adjusted frequently in response to blood glucose levels and targets, with consideration for changes in status that can increase hypoglycemia risk.

Bibliography

American Diabetes Association: Diabetes Care Executive Summary from the American Diabetes Association. Standards of medical care in diabetes 2009. *Diabetes Care.* 2009;32(suppl 1): S6–S12.

Ashraf W, Wong DT, Ronayne M, Williams D. Guidelines for preoperative administration of patients home medications. *J Perianesth Nurs.* 2004;19(4):228–233.

Braithwaite S, Buie M, Thompson C, et al. Hospital hypoglycemia: not only treatment but also prevention. *Endocr Pract.* 2004;10(suppl 2):S89–S99.

Cryer P, Axelrod L, Grossman A, et al. Evaluation and management of adult hypoglycemic disorders: an endocrine society practice guideline. *J Clin Endocrinol Metab.* 2009;94(3):709–728.

Fischer KF, Lees JA, Newman JH. Hypoglycemia in hospitalized patients: causes and outcomes. *N Engl J Med.* 1986;315(20):1245–1250.

Kitabchia A, Freire A, Umpierrez G. Evidence for strict inpatient blood glucose control: time to revise glycemic goals in hospitalized patients. *Metab Clin Exp.* 2008;57(1):116–120.

Lien LF, Bethel MA, Feinglos MN. In-hospital management of type 2 diabetes mellitus. *Med Clin N Am.* 2004;88(4):1085–1105.

Moghissi ES, Korytkowski MT, DiNardo M. American Association of Clinical Endocrinologist and American Diabetes Association consensus statement on inpatient glycemic control. *Endocr Pract.* 2009;15(4):1–17.

NICE-SUGAR Study Investigators. Intensive versus conventional glucose control in critically ill patients. *N Eng J Med.* 2009;360(13):1283–1297.

Skyler JS, Bergenstal R, Bonow RO, et al. Intensive glycemic control and the prevention of cardiovascular events: implications of the ACCORD, ADVANCE, and VA Diabetes trials. A position statement of the American Diabetes Association and a scientific statement of the American College of Cardiology Foundation and the American Heart Association. *Diabetes Care.* 2009;32(1):187–192.

Chapter 11
Transitioning to Outpatient Care

Beatrice D. Hong and Ellen D. Davis

Keywords Insulin teaching · Discharge regimen · Diabetes education · Target glucose range

Orchestrating a smooth transition to outpatient care is critical for all patients with hyperglycemia in the inpatient setting. There are many factors to consider in preparing patients for discharge. Patients need to feel comfortable with the discharge regimen; this requires both appropriate prescriptions for medications and supplies, along with patient education (Fig. 11.1).

Medication Regimen

Most patients with diabetes will be on insulin in the hospital, even if they take oral medications at home. Additionally, postoperative patients who did not have a previous diagnosis of diabetes may develop hyperglycemia and then require insulin during the admission and at discharge.

When prescribing new insulin therapy, remember to consider the following:

- Is the patient capable and willing to inject insulin at home? If not, is there a family member or caretaker who is willing to take on this responsibility?
- Will home health be necessary temporarily for follow-up education?

Consider continuation of insulin in the following patients:

Postoperative patients. Insulin is the treatment of choice in postoperative patients to allow optimal healing and reduce the risk of infections. Data supports particular use to prevent mediastinitis in patients who have undergone coronary artery bypass graft and other types of thoracic surgery.

B.D. Hong (✉)
Division of Endocrinology, Metabolism, and Nutrition, Department of Medicine, Duke University Medical Center, Durham, NC 27710, USA
e-mail: beatrice.hong@duke.edu

L.F. Lien et al. (eds.), *Glycemic Control in the Hospitalized Patient*,
DOI 10.1007/978-1-60761-006-9_11, © Springer Science+Business Media, LLC 2011

Checklist for Discharge

- Medication regimen, clearly stated
- Prescriptions for discharge: medication and supplies
- Instructions about glucose monitoring and reporting results
- Instructions for managing hyper- and hypoglycemia
- Behavior recommendations, ie diet and exercise
- Follow-up appointments

Fig. 11.1 Checklist for discharge

Large doses of insulin. Patients who require large amounts of insulin in the hospital, i.e., greater than 40 units daily, will most likely need to be discharged on insulin.

Contraindications to non-insulin antidiabetic medications. Patients who have pre-existing or newly developed contraindications to the use of non-insulin antidiabetic medications will require insulin. Some contraindications include decreased renal function, impaired liver function, pancreatitis, or congestive heart failure. A complete list of non-insulin antidiabetic medications and respective contraindications is found in Chapter 9: Non-insulin therapy.

Insulin Teaching

Often, staff nurses are able to teach patients how to manage their insulin. Some hospitals also offer special classes. Certified Diabetes Educators (CDE), when available, can assist with teaching complex regimens or patients with unique needs. Patients should have supervised, hands-on practice with injection of insulin and should be able to demonstrate proper technique prior to discharge. With appropriate advance notice, staff nurses can direct patients to self-administer scheduled insulin doses. Patients also should be able to demonstrate proper needle disposal.

Choice of Discharge Regimen

A complete guide to insulin regimens is found in Chapter 2: Subcutaneous insulin (Table 11.1). Commonly used discharge regimens are described below.

Premixed insulin regimen. The premixed insulin regimen is a two-injection daily regimen. There are various available formulations of premixed insulin; each incorporates an intermediate-acting insulin with either a short- or rapid-acting insulin. This regimen is an attractive option for patients who have very stable day-to-day activities and meals. However, this is a very limited population of patients. When used improperly, patients can have frequent hyper- and hypoglycemia.

Table 11.1 Discharge regimens

Regimen	Example	Pros	Cons	Treatment niche
Non-insulin medication	A detailed list is found in Chapter 9: Non-insulin antidiabetic medication	Some consider oral to be an easier administration route; less frequent monitoring required	Many contraindications; may not give adequate glucose control; rarely useful for patients with type 1 diabetes	Patients with type 2 diabetes who refuse insulin or who have low insulin requirements. Consider on case-by-case basis
Premixed insulin	Humulin® 70/30™ twice daily Novolin® 70/30™ twice daily NovoLog® MIX 70/30™ twice daily Humalog® MIX 75/25™ twice daily	Twice daily dosing	Inflexible component ratios make titration difficult. Not appropriate for patients with inconsistent eating. May have more fasting hyperglycemia and more frequent hypoglycemia	Limited population; requires significant education on rigidity (and potential danger) of regimen, and the need to eat 3 meals at exact times each day, with a standard carbohydrate amount
Two-injection split-mix insulin	Regular and NPH insulin (mixed), injected before breakfast + Regular and NPH insulin (mixed), injected before supper	Improved flexibility over premixed insulins because individual components can be titrated	No short-acting coverage for the noon meal. May see fasting hyperglycemia and more frequent hypoglycemia	Limited population. Consider this regimen in patients who are willing to mix insulin but who are not willing to give more than two daily injections
Three-injection split-mix insulin	Regular and NPH insulin before breakfast (mixed in a single syringe) + Regular insulin before supper + NPH at bedtime	Improved flexibility over premixed insulins because individual components can be titrated	No short-acting coverage for the noon meal. Still not as precise titration as the basal-bolus regimen	Limited population. Consider this regimen in patients who are willing to mix insulin but who are not willing to give more than three daily injections

Table 11.1 (continued)

Regimen	Example	Pros	Cons	Treatment niche
Basal-bolus insulin	Rapid-acting insulin (lispro [Humalog®], aspart [Novolog®], glulisine [Apidra®]) at mealtimes With Long-acting insulin (glargine [Lantus®], detemir [Levemir®]) at bedtime Or Regular insulin at mealtimes And NPH at bedtime	The most flexible and "physiologic" insulin regimen	Four or more daily injections and frequent monitoring	Should be recommended for most patients who require insulin; intensive education is required
Continuous subcutaneous insulin infusion (CSII)	Details of CSII can be found in Chapter 8: insulin pumps			Not appropriate for new start in the hospital

Split-mix insulin regimen. The split-mix insulin regimen is a less intensive but reasonable alternative to the basal-bolus regimen described below. It can involve two or three injections daily and typically incorporates intermediate and short-acting insulins (Table 11.1). The advantage of the split-mix regimen is improved flexibility over premixed regimens, low cost, and fewer daily injections than the gold-standard basal-bolus regimen. However, it requires that patients eat meals consistently, and patients need to be willing and able to mix insulins for administration.

Basal-bolus insulin regimen. A basal-bolus insulin regimen usually is the best choice for both optimal glycemic control and prevention of hypoglycemia. This type of regimen often incorporates one or two injections of long-acting insulin, such as glargine (Lantus®) or detemir (Levemir®), paired with mealtime injections of a rapid-acting insulin, such as aspart (Novolog®), lispro (Humalog®), or glulisine (Apidra®). These types of insulin are favored because they allow for flexibility of schedule; however they are expensive for patients who do not have insurance coverage for medication. An alternative plan incorporates use of regular insulin at mealtimes and NPH insulin at bedtime. These insulins are less expensive, but the timing of dose administration is more rigid. Appropriate use of either of these regimens requires that the patient be capable of administration of four or five insulin injections each day, as well as frequent monitoring.

In addition to any of the choices above, the patient can also be taught to use a *correctional insulin scale*, sometimes referred to as a "sliding scale." (NOTE: The correctional insulin scale is a reasonable tool when used *in addition* to the scheduled regimens above, but it should be *not* be used alone.) Consider a correctional insulin scale for patients who have a good understanding of insulin use and who need frequent adjustments in mealtime insulin dose. It is used at mealtime only and not at bedtime or in the middle of the night. For patients who are new to insulin or who are having difficulty internalizing the basics of self-management, a correctional insulin scale can be confusing and dangerous. (More information on the advantages and disadvantages of a correctional insulin scale can be found in Chapter 2: Subcutaneous Insulin.)

Upon returning home, patients' insulin requirements are likely to change with changes in activity level and diet. Communication and follow-up are critical elements of good diabetes care.

Glucose Monitoring Post-discharge and Reporting Results

All patients should have personalized instructions for the glucose monitoring strategy. Objectives of home testing are improved glycemic control and improved quality of life. Behaviors have the best chance of implementation with creation of an individualized plan.

For patients who are using insulin, the recommendation is typically for glucose monitoring four times daily, i.e., with meals and at bedtime. For patients on oral or other non-insulin medications, monitoring frequency may be less often but should not be less than daily. Some patients will need to monitor overnight (3 AM glucoses occasionally. Pregnant patients and those on continuous subcutaneous insulin infusions (CSII, "insulin pumps," Chapter 8) will need monitoring as often as six or eight times daily. In patients for whom cost or motivation is an issue, staggered monitoring may be appropriate. In this scenario, the patient tests once or twice a day, at varying times. By the end of a week, the patient will have captured readings from all important data points. For selected patients, use of this strategy can result in more data collection than an "all or none approach."

For a patient to be invested in ongoing testing, he or she needs to understand individual, short-term, measurable benefits. Asking patients to "test in pairs" can be effective. For example, a patient on rapid-acting insulin at mealtime can implement testing before and 2 h after a meal, or before and after exercise. This helps to reveal causality and can strengthen motivation.

Target Glucose Ranges

- Fasting and preprandial blood glucoses between 70 and 140 mg/dL.
- Postprandial blood glucoses < 180 mg/dL.
- For patients who are elderly or who have frequent problems with hypoglycemia, targets may not be as strict. Conversely, pregnant patients have tighter targets. An individual approach is critical, and outpatient follow-up is essential.

Recording and Reporting

Patients need to understand the importance of the patient-provided glucose data to outpatient providers. They should be encouraged to keep a written blood glucose log. Many meter kits come with a logbook; alternatively, these can be bought separately, self-made, acquired on the internet, or even graphed on the computer if desired. Depending on the clinical situation, patients may also want to include monitoring of insulin doses, carbohydrate counting, or recording of food and exercise, at least for short term or periodically.

Hypo- and Hyperglycemia

Basic instructions about hypoglycemia management are *always* appropriate, even for patients who are experienced with insulin and diabetes self-management. It is often helpful to provide specific parameters for when to call a provider for help for either hypo- or hyperglycemia, as in the sample discharge instructions in Fig. 11.2. Some patients may be able to adjust insulin based on home monitoring, and appropriate instructions should be given in this situation as well.

Prescriptions

At the time of discharge, patients should have an updated supply at home, or be given prescriptions, for the following items (Fig. 11.3):

Diabetes Discharge Instructions

Blood Glucose Testing - Test blood sugar before every meal and at bedtime or on your provider's recommended schedule. Record the glucose readings, and take this record with you to your doctor appointments.

Take your insulin as follows:

[Fill in type of insulin_____] XX units with breakfast

[Fill in type of insulin_____] XX units with lunch

[Fill in type of insulin_____] XX units with dinner

[Fill in type of insulin_____] XX units at bedtime.

Correctional insulin scale:

If your blood sugar is greater than 150 before a meal, you will need to take some extra rapid-acting insulin with your dose. Use correction insulin only at meal times. Do not add extra to your bedtime dose of long-acting insulin.

For Blood Sugar (mg/dL),	Take an additional
151 – 200	XX units of [Fill in type of insulin_____]
201 – 250	XX units of [Fill in type of insulin_____]
251 – 300	XX units of [Fill in type of insulin_____]
301 – 350	XX units of [Fill in type of insulin_____]
351 – 400	XX units of [Fill in type of insulin_____]
Over 400	XX units of [Fill in type of insulin_____]
	AND CALL YOUR DOCTOR

Hypoglycemia instructions: If your blood sugar is less than 70 mg/dL (3.8 mmol/L), treat with one of the following options: Take 3 glucose tablets, drink a ½ cup of juice or ½ can of regular soda. Recheck blood sugar in 30 minutes. Call your doctor or emergency medical services if you still have trouble getting the blood sugar to come up to 70 mg/dL or higher.

If hypoglycemia occurs when it is longer than 1 hour until your next regularly-scheduled meal or snack, follow the treatment with a mixed protein and carbohydrate food, like peanut butter and crackers.

Fig. 11.2 Sample discharge handout

If your blood sugar is below 80 mg/dL (4.4 mmol/L), take only ½ of the usual dose of insulin.

If you are asked not to eat or drink anything before a procedure or test, **do not** take rapid-acting insulin (lispro [Humalog®], aspart [Novolog®], or glulisine [Apidra®]) until you are eating again. **Do** take your full dose of long-acting insulin (glargine [Lantus®], detemir [Levemir®]).

If you see a pattern that a lot of your blood sugars are less than 80 mg/dL (4.4 mmol/L) or greater than 200 mg/dL (11.1 mmol/L), call your doctor. Your doctor may want to change your insulin prescription.

Your follow-up appointment with Dr.XXX is on XXX date at XXX time.

If you have any questions before you see your doctor, you may call XXX-XXX-XXXX.

Fig. 11.2 (continued)

Medications
- Oral or non-insulin medications if appropriate
- Insulin
  - A vial contains 1,000 units; one vial is approximately enough for 30 units/day for 30 days.
  - All pens contain 300 units; pens come in boxes of 5.
  - Insulin vials and pens should be replaced 1 month after being opened, even if they are not empty. Current bottles or pens may be kept at room temperature (above 32° F and below 86° F). Unopened insulin should be refrigerated.
- Glucose tablets or gel.
  - Glucose tablets are inexpensive, portable, and available over the counter. Three tablets contain approximately 12–15 g of carbohydrate, which is an appropriate starting point for the management of a conscious hypoglycemic episode. Patients can be instructed on the rule of "15s." Consume 15 g of carbohydrate, wait 15 min, retest, and re-treat with 15 g, if needed.
  - Other treatments for conscious hypoglycemia may also be recommended (i.e., 1/2 cup regular soda, 1/2 cup fruit juice).
- Glucagon kit, if appropriate. For proper use, the patient must live with, or near, someone who is comfortable emergently administering glucagon for unconscious hypoglycemia.

Patient's Name	Patient's Name
Glucose Testing Device	Glucose Test strips
Sig: Use as directed	Sig: Test 4-6 times a day
Disp: #1	Disp: 200
	Refills: 2 months
Dx code	Dx code
Your signature here	Your signature here
Patient's Name	Patient's Name
Regular insulin	Novolog Flex Pen
Sig: 12 units SQ tid/ac	Sig: 8 units SQ with meals
Disp: #1 vial	Disp: 5 pens (1 box)
Refills: 2 months	Refills: 2 months
Dx code	Dx code
Your signature here	Your signature here

Disp,dispense; Dx, diagnosis; Sig, signa

Fig. 11.3 Sample prescriptions

Supplies
- Glucose meter: often referred to as a "glucometer," or, more specifically, "glucose testing device" (Fig. 11.3).
- Lancets: come in boxes of 100.
- Test strips: come in containers of 50 or 100. Sufficient test strips should be prescribed to ensure availability for regular testing and in case of emergencies.
- All manufacturers and current literature recommend using warm water and soap for easier, less painful testing with lower incidence of infection. Many hospitals also do this. There are no definitive rules for when to use alcohol on fingers when testing.

- Alternate site testing (forearms and palms) generally has lower reliability than finger testing. Information about this is available on websites like www.diabetesforecast.org and can be provided at the provider's discretion.

When writing prescriptions, be sure to include diagnosis codes, which are required for insurance coverage (Fig. 11.3).

Diabetes medications and supplies may be expensive. This should be considered when choosing a regimen for discharge. The following are some tips to help patients use their money wisely.

- There is no generic insulin. Regular and NPH are the least expensive insulins at retail price. Many of the newer insulins may be available through company financial assistance programs.
- Glucose meters are often free or inexpensive, but test strips are expensive. Large chain stores may have supplies at discounted prices. Choice of brand of testing supplies is influenced by specific insurance coverage, including Medicaid.
- Advance discussion about cost of testing supplies and cost-effective testing regimens may lessen the impact of cost as a barrier to self-management.

Behavior Recommendations

Medical nutrition therapy (MNT). All patients with diabetes should receive individualized MNT as needed to achieve treatment goals. A thorough discussion of this topic can be found in Chapter 7: Medical Nutrition Therapy.

Exercise. Patients should be encouraged to engage in at least 150 min of moderate-intensity aerobic exercise per week unless exercise is contraindicated. Use of exercise prescriptions and individualized plans can be helpful.

Follow-Up Appointments

Follow-up appointments should be made within 1–2 weeks of the discharge date for patients with a new diagnosis of diabetes, with recurrent episodes of hypo- or hyperglycemia during the admission, or with major changes to the outpatient diabetes regimen.

Follow-up with an endocrinologist may also be appropriate, particularly in the following situations:

- The patient was seen by an endocrinologist while admitted, and specific follow-up is recommended.
- The patient starts a new basal-bolus insulin regimen.
- The patient has type 1 diabetes.
- The patient has frequent hypoglycemia or hypoglycemia unawareness.

Other Referrals to Consider

- Outpatient diabetes education
- Nutrition
- Diabetes support and education groups. The local American Diabetes Association (ADA) branch can provide information about these. Additionally, patients may want to utilize local community resources through their doctor's offices, churches, senior centers, etc.

Sample Discharge Instructions

Given the complexity of discharge instructions for patients with diabetes, we recommend providing a handout with personalized diabetes discharge instructions (Fig. 11.2). The handout will serve as a useful reference when diabetes self-care questions arise after discharge. The handout also will help the patient and family to focus on the key elements of diabetes management and to separate these issues from the myriad of general discharge instructions that patients are given when they leave the hospital.

Bibliography

American Association of Diabetes Educators (AADE). Inpatient position statement. http://www.diabeteseducator.org/ProfessionalResources. Accessed April 9, 2009.

American Diabetes Association. Diabetes care executive summary from the American Diabetes Association. Standards of medical care in diabetes 2010. *Diabetes Care*. 2010;(supp 1):S6–S12.

Anderson RM, Funnell MM, Burkhart N, Gillard ML, Nwankwo R. *101 Tips for Behavior Change in Diabetes Education*. Alexandria, VA: American Diabetes Association; 2002.

Boinpally T, Jovanovic L. Management of type 2 diabetes and gestational diabetes in pregnancy. Mt Sinai J Med. 2009;76(3):269–280.

Clement S, Braithwaite SS, Magee MF, et al. Management of diabetes and hyperglycemia in hospitals. *Diabetes Care*. 2004;27(2):553–591.

Davis E, Midgett L, Gourley C. Teach less, teach better at every opportunity. *Diabetes Educ*. 1994;20(3):236–240.

Leak A, Davis ED, Mabrey M, Houchin L. Diabetes self management and patient education in hospitalized oncology patients. *Clin J Oncol Nurs*. 2009;13(2):205–210.

Lien LF, Bethel MA, Feinglos MN. In-hospital management of type 2 diabetes mellitus. *Med Clin N Am*. 2004;88(4):1085–1105.

Moghissi ES, Korytkowski MT, DiNardo M. American Association of Clinical Endocrinologist and American Diabetes Association consensus statement on inpatient glycemic control. *Endocr Pract*. 2009;15(4):1–17.

Chapter 12
Management of Hyperglycemia Associated with Enteral and Parenteral Nutrition

Sarah Gauger

Keywords Enteral nutrition · Parenteral nutrition (TPN) · Continuous feeding · Bolus feeding · 10% dextrose (D10)

Understanding Enteral Nutrition

Enteral nutrition, also known as "tube feeding," is necessary for patients who cannot eat but who have an intact gastrointestinal system. This may be attributed to a variety of conditions, including altered mental status, inability to swallow, and risk for aspiration. Hyperglycemia is common after the initiation of enteral nutrition in both diabetic and nondiabetic patients because the formulas are designed to be calorically dense. Furthermore, they often are delivered continuously throughout the day rather than as discrete meals. Because the choice of formula for an individual patient incorporates a variety of factors (protein, fat, and carbohydrate content, along with micronutrients), resultant hyperglycemia generally is most appropriately managed by matching subcutaneous insulin injections to the patient's needs rather than by changing the formula to correct hyperglycemia.

When treating hyperglycemia related to enteral feeding, it is important to clarify the following three elements with the ordering provider:

1. Is the feeding continuous, bolus, or nocturnal?
2. Is it anticipated that the patient will begin eating while still on the enteral feeding?
3. What type of enteral feeding formula is being used? (Table 12.1).

There are several low-carbohydrate formulas designed for patients who have problems with hyperglycemia. For patients with persistent hyperglycemia despite use of insulin, or for those who develop erratic hypoglycemia, a nutrition consult

S. Gauger (✉)
Duke Inpatient Diabetes Management, Duke University Medical Center, Durham, NC 27710, USA
e-mail: gauge003@mc.duke.edu

L.F. Lien et al. (eds.), *Glycemic Control in the Hospitalized Patient,*
DOI 10.1007/978-1-60761-006-9_12, © Springer Science+Business Media, LLC 2011

Table 12.1 Enteral feeding formulas

Product name	Osmolite 1 Cal©	Jevity 1.2 Cal ©	Isosource® 1.5 Cal	Novasource® renal
Cal/mL	1.06	1.2	1.5	2.0
Carbohydrate source	Corn maltodextrin, corn syrup solids	Corn maltodextrin, corn syrup solids, scFOS	Maltodextrin, sugar	Corn syrup, fructose
Carbohydrate (g/L)	143.9	169.4	170	200
Carbohydrate (% Cal)	54.3	52.5	44	40
Fiber (g/L)	–	18.0	8	–

Isosource® and Novasource® are registered trademarks of Société des Produits Nestlé S.A., Vevey, Switzerland
© 2010 Abbott Laboratories. Used with permission

may be helpful to explore alternative formula solutions. Switching to a low-carbohydrate formula may not completely resolve the hyperglycemia, but it may improve the ease of insulin management.

Hyperglycemia Management

Hyperglycemia related to enteral feeding must be managed with insulin. Creation of a regimen can be tricky because of the unusual nutrition timing. A simple way to begin is to calculate a starting total daily dose of insulin. This can then be divided into appropriately timed insulin injections in accordance with the nutrition pattern (Table 12.2).

Steps for determination of a total daily dose can be found in Chapter 2: Subcutaneous Insulin. The following information must be gathered in order to make a proper dose calculation:

- Does the patient have previously diagnosed diabetes? If yes, which type?
- What medications for diabetes does the patient take at home? Has this been effective in lowering the A_{1C} to the patient's treatment goal, or are changes necessary?
- Has there been hypoglycemia in the past 24 hours?

In order to determine the timing and dosages of insulin, the following information must be obtained (Table 12.2):

- If the patient is already receiving subcutaneous insulin injections, at what time are the injections being given?
- Does the timing of the insulin injections match the timing of administration of the enteral feeding?

Table 12.2 Insulin regimens for enteral feeding

Enteral feeding regimen	Subcutaneous insulin strategy for patients with diabetes	Subcutaneous insulin strategy for patients without known diabetes	Blood Glucose Monitoring	Other notes
Continuous feeding	Regular insulin in 4 divided doses. The doses are administered every 6 h over each 24-h period	Same	At least every 6 h	
Bolus feeding – every 3 h	Regular insulin every 6 h, given 30 min before alternating tube-feed boluses	Same	With each dose of insulin. (Consider more frequent monitoring early on, i.e., with each bolus, to assess for hypoglycemia.)	An alternative strategy is to give a long-acting insulin once daily and rapid-acting insulin with each bolus, although this frequency of injection and monitoring is not as convenient
Bolus feeding – every 4 h	This is not the preferred timing strategy for tube feeding because it makes coordination with insulin difficult. Consider changing to every 3-h boluses if possible			
Nocturnal feeding (e.g., 1800–0600)	1800 (or the start of feeding): regular insulin 2100: NPH insulin, and consider an additional small dose of regular insulin for those who have overnight hyperglycemia Between 0600 and 1800 (daytime hours), when feeding is suspended, some patients will require low doses of regular insulin, given at 0600 and 1200, to prevent hyperglycemia	Insulin at 1800 and 2100 for patients with diabetes is usually sufficient. Rarely, daytime coverage is also needed	Glucose monitoring should occur prior to administration of insulin at 1800 and 2100. Monitoring at 0300, 0600, and 1200 will detect other potentially abnormal glucoses. (Once a regimen is established, the 0300 check can be discontinued.)	We describe the 1800–0600 pattern because these feeding times correspond with usual insulin administration times

Table 12.2 (continued)

Enteral feeding regimen	Subcutaneous insulin strategy for patients with diabetes	Subcutaneous insulin strategy for patients without known diabetes	Blood Glucose Monitoring	Other notes
Nocturnal feeding + eating	Similar to nocturnal feeding above. Additional regular insulin is usually needed with meals	Same	With meals, at bedtime, and at 0300	In this case the 0600 blood glucose check and the insulin dose may need to be moved to 0800 to correspond more closely with the morning meal
Total parenteral nutrition	Regular insulin every 6 h Or For selected patients, long-acting insulin once daily	Regular insulin every 6 h as needed	Every 6 h	Insulin is often added to the TPN bag, so some patients will not need additional subcutaneous insulin

- If not, then adjustments must be made so that the insulin and feeding times match. For example, if the patient is only receiving nocturnal feedings, then the amount of insulin injected during the daytime should be minimal, to avoid hypoglycemia.
- For patients receiving bolus feedings, the timing of the insulin injections and the food boluses should be coordinated. For example, if boluses are being given every 3 hours, insulin injections could be given with every other bolus, which would then consist of insulin every 6 hours.

- While the administration rate of a patient's continuous enteral nutrition is increasing toward a goal rate, the carbohydrate load will also be increasing. Thus, insulin doses will need to follow.

Hypoglycemia Management in Enteral Feeding

Hypoglycemia always is a concern for patients receiving insulin with enteral feedings. Feedings can be interrupted at any time due to problems with position or function of the tube or because feeding is paused in preparation for procedures.

The most common reason for hypoglycemia with enteral feeding is an unexpected interruption in feeding. Hypoglycemia can be treated acutely by conventional methods (see Chapter 10: Hypoglycemia). In order to prevent recurrent hypoglycemia in this situation, the patient will need prolonged carbohydrate support for the active life of the insulin that was given. If feeding cannot be reinitiated promptly, it is recommended to begin a low-dose infusion of IV dextrose (D10) until feeding is restarted or until the insulin is no longer active (see Chapter 10: Hypoglycemia, Fig. 10.3). Frequent monitoring (hourly) will determine whether more acute hypoglycemia management or carbohydrate support is needed. If hypoglycemia is not the result of a food interruption, insulin dosages should be decreased; a 10–20% reduction is reasonable.

Because hypoglycemia is common in patients receiving enteral feeding, it is advisable to take measures for prevention. At our institution, we employ the following standard orders:

- Give half of the scheduled dose of regular insulin when feeding is interrupted.

  - Patients with type 2 diabetes may have a decreased insulin requirement with prolonged fasting, and other patients may have a low nutritional insulin requirement relative to their basal needs. In those patients, even smaller doses of insulin may be given during periods of interrupted feeding. In fact, some patients with type 2 diabetes may not require any insulin during periods of fasting.
  - Patients with type 1 diabetes always should be given insulin and should be supported with IV dextrose if necessary in order to enable administration of insulin.

- Administer IV D5 or D10 as soon as any unexpected interruption of enteral feeding occurs (see Chapter 10: Hypoglycemia, Fig. 10.3).

A few patients may require administration of long-acting basal insulin during their time on enteral or parenteral nutrition. In these patients, it is important for that insulin to cover only the patient's basal needs and not the nutrition. With use of long-acting insulin, there is a high risk for profound hypoglycemia associated with unplanned discontinuation of the nutrition source. For this reason, we generally prefer shorter-acting insulins (Table 12.2).

Total Parenteral Nutrition

Total parenteral nutrition (TPN) delivers a nutritional source intravenously to patients who cannot be fed through the digestive system. Common reasons for use include bowel obstruction, pancreatitis, or Crohn's disease. Patients who develop hyperglycemia while on TPN can be managed similarly to patients on continuous enteral feeding. However, this should be done in close contact with the nutrition team, as some TPN preparations contain insulin. If the patient has additional basal and correctional insulin needs, subcutaneous or IV insulin can be used. Some patients are given simultaneous TPN and enteral or oral nutrition. For these patients, non-TPN nutritional needs should be covered with subcutaneous insulin.

In general, TPN contains 100–200 g of dextrose per bag, along with 5–20 units of regular insulin for patients with diabetes. The exact amount is determined by the nutrition team or the ordering provider and often is based on the estimate of 1 unit of insulin per 10 g of carbohydrate. Over time, the dextrose concentration of the formula is increased, and the insulin also is increased. It is not recommended to use more than 100 units of insulin per bag.

Blood glucose monitoring should be performed at least every 6 hours on all patients initiated on TPN. If there is no elevation in blood glucoses within the first 72 hours in a nondiabetic patient, it may be reasonable to discontinue monitoring. For patients who are diabetic or continue to demonstrate hyperglycemia on TPN, routine monitoring should be continued, and the patient's insulin needs can be covered with standing doses of regular insulin.

Bibliography

Clement S, Braithwaite SS, Magee MF, et al. Management of diabetes and hyperglycemia in hospitals. *Diabetes Care*. 2004;27(2):553–591.

Department of Nutrition Services, Duke University Hospital. *Adult Enteral Nutrition Formulary 2009–2011*. Durham, NC: Duke University Hospital; 2009.

Elia M, Ceriello A, Laube H, Sinclair AJ, Engfer M, Stratton RJ. Enteral nutritional support and use of diabetes-specific formulas for patients with diabetes. *Diabetes Care*. 2005;28(9):2267–2279.

McKnight KA, Carter L. From trays to tube feedings: overcoming the challenges of hospital nutrition and glycemic control. *Diabetes Spectr*. 2008;21(4):233–240.

Chapter 13
When to Consult Endocrinology

Beatrice D. Hong

Keywords Endocrinology consult

Hyperglycemia is common among hospitalized patients, and improved glycemic control has been shown to improve clinical outcomes such as infection risk and hospital length of stay (LOS). Improved glycemic control can be facilitated through a diabetes care team or general endocrinology consultation. One retrospective study examined the effect of diabetes team consultation on the outcome LOS, and the investigators reported a 56% shorter LOS among those patients who were seen by a diabetes team versus those who had no consultation.

An inpatient endocrinology consult team can assist the primary team in the diagnosis and management of hyperglycemic disorders, with the goal of optimizing patient care and, ideally, patient satisfaction as well. There are many reasons to consult endocrinology. Some situations in which an endocrinology consultation should be considered are as follows:

- Whenever there is a question about a patient's diabetes management.
- Patients with newly diagnosed diabetes mellitus of any type.
- Patients on multiple daily injections, multiple types of insulin, or large doses of insulin at home.
- Patients with type 1 diabetes mellitus.
- Patients who are pregnant.
- Patients with poor glycemic control.
- Patients with persistent hyper- or hypoglycemia, or those whose blood glucose levels fluctuate in the inpatient setting.
- Patients on continuous subcutaneous insulin infusion.
- Patients with corticosteroid-induced hyperglycemia, particularly those who have had organ transplantation.

B.D. Hong (✉)
Division of Endocrinology, Metabolism, and Nutrition, Department of Medicine, Duke University Medical Center, Durham, NC 27710, USA
e-mail: beatrice.hong@duke.edu

L.F. Lien et al. (eds.), *Glycemic Control in the Hospitalized Patient*,
DOI 10.1007/978-1-60761-006-9_13, © Springer Science+Business Media, LLC 2011

- Patients with chronic renal insufficiency, including those on hemodialysis or peritoneal dialysis.
- Patients on an IV insulin infusion, including postoperative patients.
- Patients with other types of diabetes: cystic fibrosis-related diabetes, pancreoprivic diabetes (patients with their pancreas destroyed by medical condition or surgically removed), maturity onset diabetes of the young (MODY), or latent autoimmune diabetes in adults (LADA).
- Patients with hypoglycemia unawareness.
- Patients with complicated nutrition regimens, including those on enteral or parenteral nutrition.

Bibliography

Furnary A, Gao G, Grunkemeier G, et al. Continuous insulin infusion reduces mortality in patients with diabetes undergoing coronary artery bypass grafting. *J Thorac Cardiovasc Surg* 2003;125(5):1007–1021.

Furnary A, Wu Y, Bookin S. Effect of hyperglycemia and continuous intravenous insulin infusions on outcomes of cardiac surgical procedures: the Portland Diabetic Project. *Endocr Pract.* 2004;10(suppl 2):21–33.

Levetan C, Salas J, Wilets I. Impact of endocrine and diabetes team consultation on hospital length of stay for patients with diabetes. *Am J Med.* 1995;99:22–28.

Lien L, Bethel M, Feinglos M. In-hospital management of type 2 diabetes mellitus. *Med Clin N Am.* 2004;88(4):1085–1105.

Chapter 14
Frequently Asked Questions

Mary E. Cox and Matthew J. Crowley

Keywords Hypoglycemia · Basal insulin · Prandial insulin · Plasma glucose · Point-of-care glucose · Correction dose insulin · Non-insulin antidiabetic medication · Abnormal glucose measurement

Many questions come through the diabetes management service pager at our institution. This chapter discusses some frequently asked questions and recommended strategies for management of common situations. This discussion provides focused recommendations; further details about many topics can be found in their respective chapters.

Definitions

- *Plasma glucose*: Glucose can be measured in plasma and used to diagnose diabetes. In the hospital, plasma glucose measurements often are used to confirm a reading obtained by a point-of-care glucose meter. Plasma testing is generally the most reliable option for measuring blood glucose.
- *Point-of-care glucose monitoring*: A point-of-care glucose meter, also known as a glucometer or capillary glucose monitor, can be used to measure whole blood glucose. Point-of-care testing (POCT) often is used in the hospital to make real-time decisions about therapy. In general, the accuracy of these meters is good, and they are calibrated to reflect the plasma glucose; however, they may be limited at particularly high or low glucose levels.
- *Hypoglycemia*: Hypoglycemia typically is defined as plasma or blood glucose less than 70 mg/dL (3.8 mmol/L); in our institution, a documented glucose below this level automatically activates an inpatient "hypoglycemia protocol," with instructions to verify the measurement and administer 50% dextrose (D50) as indicated. Of note, some patients without diabetes, especially young women, may have normal fasting glucose levels below 60 mg/dL (3.3 mmol/L). This is

M.E. Cox (✉)
Division of Endocrinology, Metabolism, and Nutrition, Department of Medicine, Duke University Medical Center, Durham, NC 27710, USA
e-mail: marybethcoxmd@gmail.com

L.F. Lien et al. (eds.), *Glycemic Control in the Hospitalized Patient*,
DOI 10.1007/978-1-60761-006-9_14, © Springer Science+Business Media, LLC 2011

not likely to be the case for most inpatients with diabetes, and any glucose below 70 mg/dL (3.8 mmol/L) in the hospital setting requires immediate attention.

- *Basal insulin*: This is a long- or intermediate-acting insulin given to control blood glucose in the fasting state. Examples include the long-acting insulins glargine (Lantus®) or detemir (Levemir®) and the intermediate-acting insulin NPH (Humulin®-NPH, Novolin® N). Basal insulin also can be provided via continuous subcutaneous insulin infusion (CSII) using aspart (Novolog®) or lispro (Humalog®).
- *Prandial insulin*: This is a short- or rapid-acting insulin given before or with meals to control rises in blood glucose that result from carbohydrate ingestion. Timing of prandial insulin administration is dependent on the timing of carbohydrate exposure. Carbohydrate sources include oral intake, other enteral nutrition, and total parenteral nutrition (TPN). Regular insulin (Novolin® R, Humulin® R) is the most common short-acting type; because onset of activity occurs at approximately 30 min after injection, regular insulin should be given 30 min before a meal. Available rapid-acting insulins include aspart (Novolog®), lispro (Humalog®), and glulisine (Apidra®); onset of activity occurs at approximately 5–15 min after injection, so these insulins can be given with or just after meals. Prandial insulin is sometimes referred to as "bolus" insulin.
- *Correction dose insulin*: This short- or rapid-acting insulin is given in addition to scheduled insulin for the purpose of correcting hyperglycemia.
- *Non-insulin antidiabetic medications*: These medications include oral and injectable medications other than insulin.

Abnormal Glucose Measurements
How Do I Manage Hypoglycemia in Hospitalized Patients?

If a hypoglycemic patient exhibits severe neuroglycopenic symptoms such as altered mental status, coma, or seizure, immediately administer 1 ampule of D50 intravenously and provide appropriate symptomatic treatment and frequent glucose monitoring. For all asymptomatic patients or patients with less severe symptoms such as tremor, palpitations, anxiety, sweating, hunger, or paresthesias, proceed with the following steps for confirmation and treatment:

1. Repeat the glucose measurement for confirmation. A repeat POCT glucose can be done quickly, but sometimes it also is useful to obtain a plasma glucose measurement, particularly in patients who are asymptomatic. Some patients do have true hypoglycemia without symptoms, so treatment should not be delayed while waiting for a confirmatory plasma measurement.
2. Determine the patient's access route for glucose administration. The oral route is preferred if the patient is awake and alert. Glucose also can be administered intravenously, intramuscularly, and through an endotracheal tube. If no access is available, give 1 mg glucagon intramuscularly (last resort).

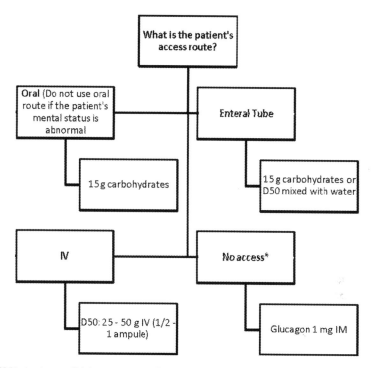

D50, 50% dextrose; IV, intravenous; IM, intramuscular.

*If a patient does not have access, this should be discussed promptly with the care team. Source: Duke University Hospital Glycemic Safety Committee, courtesy of Mary Jane Stillwagon, BSN, RN.

Fig. 14.1 Hypoglycemia algorithm. Decision about therapy should be based on the patient's mental status and access routes, using the least invasive method available. *D50*, 50% dextrose; *IV*, intravenous; *IM*, intramuscular. *If a patient does not have access, this should be discussed promptly with the care team. Source: Duke University Hospital Glycemic Safety Committee, courtesy of Mary Jane Stillwagon, BSN, RN

3. Treat the hypoglycemia (Fig. 14.1). Consider the "rule of 15s." Fifteen grams of oral carbohydrate will raise the blood glucose approximately 15 mg/dL in approximately 15 min. Of note, the glucose may continue to rise after the first 15 min by as much as 40 mg/dL. Accordingly, when treating a patient for whom oral intake is safe, start treatment with administration of 15 g of carbohydrate by mouth, understanding that the individual patient's response may vary. Oral options that provide 15 g of carbohydrates include

- 4 oz fruit juice or regular soda (1/2 cup).
- 1 packet of glucose gel
- 3–4 glucose tablets

Foods with high glucose content (as opposed to fructose or other simple sugars) are preferred. Foods with high fat content, such as ice cream or peanut butter, will not raise blood glucose as quickly because fat slows glucose absorption.

Some patients will continue to experience symptoms of tremor, headache, nausea, sweating, and food craving for 20–30 min after effective treatment. Reassurance can be helpful, concurrent with close monitoring. Resolution of symptoms is an important treatment goal, but it is important to remember that excessive amounts of carbohydrate can lead to severe rebound hyperglycemia.

4. Measure POCT glucose again 15–20 min after initial treatment. If the blood glucose level remains below 70 mg/dL (3.8 mmol/L), return to the algorithm and re-treat. Repeat the process until the glucose level is greater than 70 mg/dL (3.8 mmol/L).
5. If the blood glucose remains less than 70 mg/dL (3.8 mmo/L) after three treatments, consider a continuous infusion of 10% dextrose (D10).
6. Consider the differential diagnosis for in-hospital hypoglycemia (Table 14.1) and give special consideration to insulin and other medications. Adjustments to the patient's insulin likely will be required.
7. Once hypoglycemia is resolved, consider giving the patient a snack with mixed carbohydrate, fat, and protein content, such as peanut butter or cheese with crackers, to maintain normoglycemia until the insulin or hypoglycemic medication is metabolized.
8. Continue subsequent glucose monitoring. After an episode of hypoglycemia, it is prudent to increase the monitoring frequency until stability is assured.

Table 14.1 Causes of hypoglycemia in the hospitalized patient

- Acute or intermittent hypoglycemia
  - Excessive basal or prandial insulin doses
  - Acute renal failure
  - Acute hepatic failure
  - Infection
  - NPO status or change in nutrition pattern
  - Changing dosages of corticosteroids
  - Shock
- Persistent hypoglycemia
  - Malignancy
  - Alimentary disease
  - Adrenal insufficiency
  - Pregnancy
  - Burns

NPO, nothing by mouth

How Do I Manage Hyperglycemia in Hospitalized Patients?

Hyperglycemia is a frequent finding in hospitalized patients. There are a number of different causes (Table 14.2). Confirmation and treatment differ somewhat between patients who have a previous diagnosis of diabetes and those who do not.

Table 14.2 Causes of hyperglycemia in the hospitalized patient

- Diabetes mellitus (diagnosed or previously undiagnosed)
- Postoperative stress
- Infection
- Other inflammatory states (e.g., myocardial infarction)
- Medication side effects (e.g., corticosteroids, calcineurin inhibitors, atypical antipsychotic agents)
- Enteral or parenteral nutrition
- Vasopressor administration
- Continuous veno-venous hemodialysis

Patients Previously Diagnosed with Diabetes

The first step for management of patients with diabetes is a careful disease history, which should include the type of diabetes, the date and circumstances of the diagnosis, prior management, and importantly, the patient's current home diabetes medication regimen. Once this has been ascertained, the next step is to determine whether the home regimen should be continued during the hospital stay. To aid this decision making, it usually is helpful to obtain a hemoglobin A_{1C} as a measure of recent glycemic control (see Chapter 4: Laboratory Testing), as well as history of recent medication self-adjustments and adherence.

If the patient is taking non-insulin antidiabetic medications at home, it is generally prudent to replace them with scheduled insulin while the patient is in the hospital (see Chapter 9: Non-insulin Antidiabetic Medications). Many individuals already using scheduled insulin prior to admission will require adjustments while in the hospital (see Chapter 2: Subcutaneous Insulin).

When calculating subcutaneous insulin dosing in the hospital, a general rule is to use the following formula:

$$\text{Weight (kg)} \times X \text{ units/kg} = \text{Total daily dose(units)}$$

In this formula, $X = 0.3–0.5$ units/kg for patients with type 1 diabetes and $X = 0.5–1.0$ units/kg for patients with type 2 diabetes. Lower units per kilogram values should be used for patients who are sensitive to insulin and higher values should be used for insulin-resistant patients (see Chapter 2: Subcutaneous Insulin). If uncertainty exists about a patient's level of insulin resistance, a general recommendation is to start with a lower total daily dose (TDD) and then to promptly adjust according to subsequent POCT glucose levels.

Although correction dose insulin alone sometimes is used to treat mild or intermittent hyperglycemia, this practice should be discouraged, as scheduled insulin is known to maintain normoglycemia more effectively.

Patients Not Previously Diagnosed with Diabetes

The first step in this situation should be to confirm that the patient has not been diagnosed with diabetes mellitus. If the patient does have known diabetes, document this in the chart and proceed with treatment as per the previous section.

If the hyperglycemic patient has not been previously diagnosed with diabetes, the next step should be to determine a scheduled insulin regimen. Although correction dose insulin, sometimes referred to as "sliding scale insulin," *alone* is sometimes implemented in this situation, this practice should be discouraged. The American Diabetes Association recommends use of correction dose insulin only when given *in addition* to a scheduled insulin regimen, as the preferred method of addressing unexpected hyperglycemia. Scheduled insulin is preferred for the following reasons:

- Correction dose insulin alone is less effective than a scheduled insulin regimen in controlling hyperglycemia and decreasing hospital length of stay.
- Correction dose insulin alone does not prevent hyperglycemia.
- Correction dose insulin alone can lead to erratic glycemic control with episodes of hyperglycemia alternating with hypoglycemia.

Newly diagnosed patients with diabetes, patients who have had surgery, patients starting hyperglycemia-inducing medications, and patients with medication changes all may require continuation of insulin or other diabetes medications at hospital discharge. For these patients, inpatient education is crucial and should be arranged prior to discharge (see Chapter 11: Transition to Outpatient Care).

What if My Patient Has Severe Hyperglycemia (Glucose >400 mg/dL [>22.2 mmol/L])?

As with other POCT glucose abnormalities, it is useful to confirm an initial measurement with another POCT measurement or a plasma glucose level. If the glucose is truly elevated, assess for diabetic ketoacidosis (DKA). A simple, rapid screening test for ketoacidosis is a semi-quantitative urine ketone measurement on a routine urinalysis. If urine ketones are present, confirmatory testing should be ordered: basic metabolic panel, calculated anion gap, serum ketone level, and other appropriate testing (see Chapter 6: Hyperglycemic Emergencies). If DKA is present, initiation of an IV insulin infusion and other acute management is indicated.

For a patient with severe hyperglycemia without DKA, it is reasonable to treat with an insulin infusion, as this strategy will rapidly and accurately correct the hyperglycemia. In many hospitals, intensive monitoring and/or IV insulin infusion may require placement in an intermediate or intensive care unit. Indications for IV insulin infusion are discussed in detail in Chapter 3.

If an insulin infusion is felt not to be indicated, subcutaneous insulin should be used to correct the hyperglycemia in one of two ways, depending on whether the patient is able to eat. In both cases, a scheduled basal insulin dose should be provided. In patients for whom eating is not contraindicated, the first option is to give short- or rapid-acting insulin along with a mixed macronutrient snack or meal. If eating is contraindicated, the second option is to cautiously give short- or rapid-acting insulin without food. With the latter option, the patient's glucose should be checked every 30–60 min after insulin administration in order to assure that the glucose does not decrease more rapidly or to a greater degree than desired. Additional insulin should not necessarily be given in response to these follow-up glucose levels. Like all drugs, insulins have distinct half-lives, approximately 4–5 h for rapid-acting analogs. Repeat dosing at intervals shorter than this can cause a phenomenon called "insulin stacking," which can lead to hypoglycemia and should be avoided. If the glucose is not decreasing as expected on repeat monitoring, use of IV insulin should be reconsidered. A correction dose insulin scale can be a useful *adjunct* to scheduled subcutaneous insulin.

What if My Patient's POCT and Plasma Glucose Readings Don't Agree?

As with all laboratory tests, plasma glucose and POCT are not without error. For plasma glucose testing, expected error is approximately 20–40 mg/dL (1.1–2.2 mmol/L), and the expected error for POCT is even greater, particularly at extremes of blood glucose. Furthermore, glucose levels fluctuate within individuals over time, so levels that are not drawn simultaneously can differ. However, sometimes differences between plasma and point-of-care glucose values cannot be explained by error or time fluctuation. The following sections discuss possible explanations for true differences between POCT and plasma glucose testing.

POCT Glucose Is Lower Than Plasma Glucose

Falsely low point-of-care glucose values usually result from inaccurate measurement due to either provider or patient factors such as the following:

- Incorrect use of meter, including inadequate meter calibration, use of expired or incorrect test strip, poor technique in performing finger prick or applying blood to test strip
- Situations that cause decreased blood flow to the fingertips, such as Raynaud's phenomenon and vasopressor use
- Thickened skin, as for patients with scleroderma or calciphylaxis

Falsely elevated plasma glucoses also can occur in the following situations:

- Low hematocrit
- Hyperbilirubinemia
- Severe lipemia
- Shock and dehydration (may either lower or elevate result)
- Hypoxia (may either lower or elevate result)
- Drugs: acetaminophen overdose, ascorbic acid, dopamine, fluorescein, mannitol, and salicylates (may either lower or elevate result)

POCT Glucose Is Higher Than Plasma Glucose

Falsely elevated POCT glucose may occur due to the following:

- Caution should be used in patients on peritoneal dialysis or in those receiving therapeutic immunoglobulin preparations. Many POCT testing kits employ the chemical glucose dehydrogenase pyrroloquinoline quinone (GDH-PQQ) to quantify glucose. GDH-PQQ reacts with several non-glucose sugars, including maltose, galactose, and xylose, which are found in peritoneal dialysis solutions and therapeutic immunoglobulin preparations. Use of these testing kits in combination with use of products containing non-glucose sugars can result in a falsely elevated POCT glucose value. The US Food and Drug Administration (FDA) has released a Public Health Notification that provides a list of GDH-PQQ glucose test strips; this can be accessed at http://www.fda.gov/MedicalDevices/Safety/AlertsandNotices/PublicHealthNotifications/. In cases where it is not possible to avoid test strips that contain GDH-PQQ, errors can be avoided by use of plasma glucose. This is particularly important for elevated glucose values or those that are inconsistent with a patient's history or glucose pattern.
- Hematocrit level can affect the precision of POCT glucose (see Chapter 4: Lab Testing).

Falsely low plasma glucose may be due to the following:

- Capture of an accurate serum glucose value depends on the prompt processing of the sample, as glycolysis continues to occur in collected blood. This is a problem particularly in patients with elevated white cell counts; in these patients, the glucose can drop quite quickly in the tube. In refrigerated specimens with the preservative lithium heparin, significant changes in measured glucose should not occur before 8 h. However, this time is shortened when specimens sit at room temperature.
- High hematocrit
- Shock and dehydration (may either lower or elevate result)
- Hypoxia (may either lower or elevate result)

- Drugs: acetaminophen overdose, ascorbic acid, dopamine, fluorescein, mannitol, and salicylates (may either lower or elevate result)

Medication Timing and Administration

Incorrect use of insulin and oral diabetes medications is a common source of medication error in hospitalized patients. In order to prescribe these medications safely, it is important to become acquainted with the pharmacokinetics of each type of insulin and appropriate indications for in-hospital use of non-insulin antidiabetic medications (see Chapter 1, 2, and 9). The following are common questions regarding diabetes medication timing and administration:

What if My Patient's Diabetes Medication Is Not on My Hospital's Formulary?

In general, if a non-insulin medication is not on a hospital's formulary, it is appropriate to discontinue that agent during the hospital stay and initiate scheduled insulin. Patients taking insulin at home also often require regimen modifications or substitutions (Table 14.3). This is especially true for patients who use premixed insulin preparations, such as 70/30 insulin. Because use of premixed insulin requires stable food intake, patients using these insulins will usually benefit from transition to a basal/prandial regimen while in the hospital where food intake is often erratic (see Chapter 2: Subcutaneous Insulin)

Table 14.3 Insulin half-lives and substitutions

Insulin	Approximate half-life, h	Options for substitution
Aspart (Novolog®)	2–4	Lispro, glulisine
Lispro (Humalog®)	2–4	Aspart, glulisine
Glulisine (Apidra®)	2–4	Aspart, lispro
Regular (Novolin® R, Humulin® R)	4–6	Aspart, lispro, or glulisine, with caution
NPH (Novolin® N, Humulin® N)	10–14	Detemir, with caution
Detemir (Levemir®)	16–20	NPH or glargine
Glargine (Lantus®)	24	Detemir

What Is the Difference Between Humalog® and Humulin® or Novolog® and Novolin® Insulins?

Humulin® and Novolin® are brand names that refer to several different insulin preparations. For example, there are Humulin® Regular and Humulin® NPH insulins, as well as Novolin® Regular and Novolin® NPH insulins. Humalog®

and Novolog® are also brand names. Each corresponds to a single rapid-acting insulin analog, insulin lispro and insulin aspart, respectively.

It is important to note that many premixed insulin preparations carry the same brand names as the insulin preparations just listed, along with a number to indicate the component percentages. For example, Humalog® Mix 75/25™ and Novolog® Mix 70/30™ are not the same as Humalog® and Novolog®. Humalog® Mix 75/25™ contains 25% lispro (Humalog®), along with 75% lispro protamine, an NPH equivalent. Novolog® Mix 70/30™ contains 30% aspart (Novolog®), along with 70% aspart protamine, an NPH equivalent.

What if My Patient Wants to Manage His or Her Diabetes in the Hospital?

There are some situations where patient self-management of diabetes is appropriate in the hospital. This often includes patients on continuous subcutaneous insulin infusion (CSII) as described in detail in Chapter 8: Insulin Pumps and Glucose Sensors in the Hospital. Prerequisite patient characteristics for successful self-management should include the following:

- Motivated to self-manage
- Stable level of consciousness (usually excludes patients undergoing surgical procedures until they are stable postoperatively)
- Stable insulin requirement
- History of successfully managing diabetes at home
- Availability of necessary equipment in the hospital

When considering allowing in-hospital self-management, providers should review hospital policy and follow patient glucose levels and insulin administration closely.

My Patient Received a Full Dose of an Antidiabetic Medication, But Now Is Not Eating (or Enteral Feeds Have Been Held). What Should I Do?

Patient status can fluctuate rapidly during a hospitalization, and nutritional status may change at any time. Not infrequently, changes in nutritional status occur after a dose of insulin or non-insulin medication intended to cover a meal or enteral feeding has already been administered. Risk for hypoglycemia increases significantly in this situation, and action must be taken to prevent dangerous decreases in blood glucose:

- Blood glucose, patient symptoms, and vital signs should be closely monitored.
- POCT should be performed every 30–60 min for the duration of the medication's half-life.

- Patients should be advised to alert the nursing staff if any symptoms of hypoglycemia develop.
- Hypoglycemia should be treated accordingly per hospital protocol or the algorithm in Fig. 14.1.
- If the procedure cannot be delayed, it is appropriate to administer D10 (our institution utilizes an IV D10 protocol. See Chapter 10: Hypoglycemia, Fig. 10.2).
- Appropriate supervision should be ensured if patients are leaving the unit for a test or procedure before the risk for hypoglycemia has subsided.

Unexpected interruption of nutrition is the primary reason why non-insulin medications usually should be replaced by insulin at the time of hospitalization. Insulin has more predictable pharmacokinetics in hospitalized patients and is more easily adjusted to prevent hypoglycemia in these circumstances.

What if My Patient's Nutrition Regimen Changes?

Circumstances often necessitate changes in nutrition plans for hospitalized patients. For example, patients may be changed from oral intake to enteral feeding, or from continuous enteral feeding to nocturnal feeding with oral intake during the day. This scenario always calls for a review of insulin dosing (see Chapter 12: Enteral and Parenteral Nutrition).

- Calculate your patient's TDD of insulin.
- Redistribute the TDD as appropriate for the new nutrition pattern, using basal and prandial insulin as indicated.
- It may be reasonable to continue the basal insulin dose, while redistributing prandial doses to cover the new feeding pattern.

My Patient Missed a Dose of a Diabetes Medication. Should It Be Given Late?

Insulin

When an insulin dose is missed or delayed, it is important to consider the insulin type when deciding whether to administer the medication after the scheduled time.

- Basal insulin generally can be given up to a few hours late without grave consequence. Remember to consider the late administration time when analyzing the patient's blood glucose control the next day.
- Prandial insulin must be given with food, except in certain situations (see the section on the patient with severe hyperglycemia). If a patient has taken a meal without receiving scheduled insulin and more than 90 min have passed, it is best to defer prandial insulin until the next meal. It may be necessary to give correctional insulin along with the next scheduled prandial dose. If a patient with type 1 diabetes misses a prandial insulin dose, ensure that the patient has received

appropriate basal insulin; these patients must have exogenous insulin active at all times in order to avoid DKA.

Non-insulin Antidiabetic Medications

For oral antidiabetic agents that are given without relation to food intake, such as biguanides or sulfonylureas, a short delay in administration is relatively inconsequential. These medications may be given safely up to a few hours after their intended administration time. The same is not true for medications that are intended to be given before meals, such as repaglinide (Prandin®), nateglinide (Starlix®), and exenatide (Byetta®). These medications should be treated like prandial insulin. For these medications, missed doses should not be given late, but should be administered at the next scheduled dose time. (See Chapter 9: Non-insulin Antidiabetic Medications.)

What if My Patient Has Overdosed on a Diabetes Medication?

Patients sometimes present to the hospital following an intentional or unintentional overdose of insulin or other antidiabetic medication. The most common toxicity associated with this situation is hypoglycemia. (Chapter 9: Table 9.2: Non-insulin Antidiabetic Medications and Toxicities.) When managing a patient who has overdosed on a diabetes medication, consider the following:

- Treatment of overdose-induced hypoglycemia is generally symptomatic and supportive. However, if hypoglycemia is severe, action should be taken without delay (see Chapter 10: Hypoglycemia).
- Blood glucose should be monitored every 30–60 min for as long as the medication is active.
- Advise the patient to alert staff if he or she should experience symptoms of hypoglycemia such as sweating, palpitations, or tremor.
- Nurses should monitor for changes in mental status and vital signs.

Should I Give a Dose of Insulin or Non-insulin Antidiabetic Medication When . . .?

The Glucose Is in the Lower End of the Normal Range

As stated previously, hospitalized patients with diabetes or sustained hyperglycemia should receive scheduled insulin. Scheduled insulin regimens are designed to maintain normoglycemia and prevent hyperglycemia, not solely to treat blood glucose values that are already high. Thus, a normal blood sugar, even if in the lower end of the normal range, is not a valid reason to hold an insulin dose. If a patient exhibits a persistent pattern of blood glucose values below the desired range, the entire insulin regimen should be reviewed and adjusted appropriately. A blood glucose value that is truly low should result in omission or adjustment of the scheduled insulin dose.

The Patient Is Not Eating in Anticipation of a Test or Procedure

Non-insulin antidiabetic medications should be discontinued when a patient is not eating. If a patient is on a basal/bolus insulin regimen, basal insulin should be continued while the patient is not eating. If prandial (bolus) coverage is provided by rapid-acting insulin, it should be held while the patient is not eating. If prandial coverage is provided by short-acting insulin, such as regular insulin, the dose may need to be cut in half rather than held (see Chapter 10: Hypoglycemia, Table 14.2).

If a patient receiving continuous enteral tube feedings is treated with subcutaneous regular insulin every 6 h, then half of the regular insulin dose should be given, as the regular insulin provides both basal and prandial coverage under this regimen (Chapter 12: Enteral and Parenteral Nutrition).

The Insulin Dose Seems Like Too Much or Not Enough

Any time a scheduled insulin dose or insulin regimen doesn't seem to "make sense," it is reasonable to pause and reconsider. Think about the factors that affect a patient's insulin requirement, including weight, insulin sensitivity, age, comorbidities, and so on. A quick assessment of the effectiveness of previous insulin doses can be an excellent guide for whether an insulin dose is appropriate. If this is not available, recalculate the patient's weight-based dose as described in the previous section on hyperglycemia.

What Is U-500 Insulin?

Nearly all insulin preparations are sold in a standard concentration: 1 mL of solution contains 100 units of insulin (100 units/mL). This is known as "U-100" insulin. "U-500" insulin is an alternative preparation of regular insulin (Humulin® R) that contains 500 units/mL rather than the standard 100 units/mL. Many hospitals do not permit the use of U-500 insulin because of the risk for medication error, and we recommend consultation with an endocrinologist before considering its use.

Hardware Malfunction

"Hardware" refers to tubes and catheters used for food and medication administration. It is important to be familiar with some of the most common malfunctions that can affect diabetes management.

What if an IV Insulin Infusion Is Not Lowering the Blood Glucose as Expected?

An apparently ineffective insulin infusion may result from problems with any part of the infusion apparatus, from an infiltrated IV catheter to an empty insulin reservoir. Review the following steps:

- Check to assure that the IV catheter has not been infiltrated.
- Check tubing for leaks and faulty connections.
- Check the insulin reservoir to assure that it is not empty or connected to the wrong tubing. It may be necessary to request a new insulin reservoir from the pharmacy, as occasionally medication bags may be incorrectly labeled or contain an incorrect substance.
- Check to assure that the pump is plugged in and that the rate is set appropriately.

If all of these items are functioning correctly, continue to follow the insulin infusion protocol, and discuss the case with an endocrinologist. Extreme insulin resistance states can sometimes be refractory to even high-dose IV insulin, and this situation is best managed with endocrinology assistance.

My Patient's Feeding Tube Is Clogged and Enteral Nutrition Is Being Interrupted. What Should I Do About the Insulin?

Insulin management in this situation depends on the prescribed insulin regimen:

- If the patient is on a basal/bolus insulin regimen, the basal insulin component can be continued while the patient is not receiving enteral nutrition. The bolus insulin should be discontinued.
- If a patient receiving continuous enteral tube feedings is treated with subcutaneous regular insulin every 6 h, half of the regular insulin dose should be given, as the regular insulin provides both basal and prandial coverage under this regimen.
- Our institution uses an IV D10 infusion protocol when enteral feedings are discontinued unexpectedly after insulin has been given (see Chapter 10: Hypoglycemia, Fig. 10.2).

What if My Patient's Insulin Pump Malfunctions in the Hospital?

The inpatient strategy for this situation is simple: The CSII should be discontinued and the insulin pump removed, and scheduled subcutaneous insulin should be initiated. The patient or patient's family should call the help number on the back of the pump before discharge so that equipment problems can be corrected. This ensures that CSII can be restarted in a timely manner. To safely convert a patient from an insulin pump to an appropriate subcutaneous insulin regimen, use the CSII parameters as a guide (see Chapter 8: Insulin Pumps, for a detailed discussion):

- The total daily basal insulin dose from pump can be given as a single long-acting insulin dose. It takes several hours for long-acting insulins like glargine and levemir to take effect, so ensure that the patient has adequate insulin coverage in the meantime.
- The insulin-to-carbohydrate ratio from the insulin pump can be converted to a short- or rapid-acting prandial insulin injection. The patient should count carbohydrates as with CSII to determine an appropriate dose.

- The patient's insulin sensitivity factor (ISF) can be converted to correctional insulin. The ISF represents the decrease in plasma glucose that occurs with 1 unit of insulin. For example, an ISF of 50 indicates that 1 unit of insulin will decrease the glucose by 50 mg/dL (2.7 mmol/L). Correctional insulin for this patient with an ISF of 50 would be a scale of 1 additional unit for each 50 mg/dL (2.7 mmol/L) greater than 150 mg/dL (98.3 mmol/L). Alternatively, 5% of the TDD of scheduled insulin can be used as the increment for the correctional insulin scale (see Chapter 2: Subcutaneous Insulin).

Special Situations

What if My Pregnant Patient with Diabetes Goes into Labor?

The process of labor and delivery presents a challenge to maintenance of blood glucose control. The following points should be kept in mind when caring for patients with diabetes entering labor:

- If the patient has type 1 diabetes, consider an IV insulin infusion, and call an endocrinologist for help.
- In patients with type 2 or gestational diabetes, insulin requirements generally decrease during and immediately following labor. Consider an IV insulin infusion; if using subcutaneous insulin, be ready to decrease doses accordingly.
- Insulin decreases are usually required for peripartum patients with type 1 diabetes, as well. In these patients, balance the potential decreased insulin requirement with avoidance of DKA; this is most safely and easily accomplished with an IV insulin infusion.
- For patients with type 2 diabetes that were not on insulin prior to pregnancy, it may be acceptable to hold insulin during labor and delivery, and follow the glucoses postpartum to determine whether a subcutaneous regimen is needed.
- For patients on insulin prior to the pregnancy, resume prepregnancy doses immediately postpartum. Monitoring glucose frequently (7–8 times daily) is critically important during this period of glucose management and insulin adjustment.
- Breastfeeding can lower a patient's insulin requirement, and should prompt close glucose monitoring.

What if My Patient Has an Insulin Allergy?

Often the insulin "allergy" is a skin reaction to insulin that is injected incorrectly. Ask the staff nurse to review insulin injection with the patient. If this is not the case, and the patient truly appears to be allergic to insulin, you must consult endocrinology for assistance.

Questions from Outpatients

Diabetes-related phone calls from outpatients occur frequently. The following are situations that should be dealt with immediately:

What Should I Do When My Hyperglycemic Patient Has Positive Urine Ketones?

Many patients with type 1 or ketosis-prone type 2 diabetes have urine ketone test strips at home, and know to test their urine for ketones when hyperglycemic. If a hyperglycemic patient has ketonuria, this generally warrants a trip to the emergency room. Selected patients can be managed from home if they are able to eat and drink, but this should be done under the supervision of an endocrinologist. Patients without access to ketone strips who are experiencing persistent nausea, vomiting, and abdominal pain in the setting of hyperglycemia should proceed to the emergency room.

What Should I Do if My Patient Calls with Hypoglycemia?

If at any time a patient exhibits neuroglycopenic symptoms such as altered mental status, coma, or seizure, immediately call 911. If the hypoglycemic outpatient is unable to take anything by mouth, a family member should use a glucagon emergency injection kit if available. Otherwise, recommend immediate treatment with 15 g carbohydrates (see "Hypoglycemia" section). After treatment, repeat the glucose measurement in 15–20 min. If the patient remains hypoglycemic, re-treat, recheck, and repeat until the blood glucose is above 70. If the glucose remains below 70 after three treatments, consider calling 911, especially if the patient's mental status worsens at any time. If the patient is able to safely resolve mild hypoglycemia at home, recommend a small snack with mixed carbohydrate, fat, and protein content, such as cheese with crackers, to maintain normoglycemia. Discuss the medication regimen with the patient or a family member in order to ascertain the cause for the hypoglycemic episode, and determine whether insulin or other medications need to be changed or discontinued. If a cause for the hypoglycemia cannot be determined or if it recurs, the patient must be evaluated immediately (see Chapter 10: Hypoglycemia).

What Should I Do if My Patient's Insulin Pump Malfunctions at Home?

Ideally, patients on CSII should have a supply of backup subcutaneous insulin, with needles, syringes, and a plan for use in the event of equipment failure. If not, make immediate pharmacy arrangements for insulin and supplies, and work with the patient to compose a temporary subcutaneous insulin plan (see "What if my patient's insulin pump malfunctions in the hospital?" section above and Chapter 8). If the patient is hyperglycemic, recommend that he or she check for urine ketones as above and refer to the emergency room if indicated. The patient also should call the pump manufacturer (the phone number is on the back of the pump) and request a replacement immediately. Manufacturers often will send replacements by overnight mail.

Bibliography

Bode BW, Braithwaite SS, Steed RD, Davidson PC. Intravenous insulin infusion therapy: indications, methods, and transition to subcutaneous insulin therapy. *Endocr Pract.* 2004;10(suppl 2): 71–80.

Braithwaite S, Buie M, Thompson C, et al. Hospital hypoglycemia: not only treatment but also prevention. *Endocr Pract.* 2004;10(suppl 2):89–99.

Clement S, Braithwaite SS, Magee MF, et al. American Diabetes Association Diabetes in Hospitals Writing Committee. Management of diabetes and hyperglycemia in hospitals. *Diabetes Care.* 2004;27(2):553–591.

Cochran E, Musso E, Gorden P. The use of U-500 in patients with extreme insulin resistance. *Diabetes Care.* 2005;28(5):1240–1244.

Cryer P, Axelrod L, Grossman A, et al. Evaluation and management of adult hypoglycemic disorders: an endocrine society practice guideline. *J Clin Endocrinol Metab.* 2009;94(3):709–728.

Davidson P, Hebblewhite H, Steed R, Bode B. Analysis of guidelines for basal-bolus insulin dosing: basal insulin, correction factor, and carbohydrate-to-insulin ratio. *Endocr Pract.* 2008;14(9):1095–1101.

Fischer KF, Lees JA, Newman JH. Hypoglycemia in hospitalized patients: causes and outcomes. *N Engl J Med.* 1986;315(20):1245–1250.

Hirsch I, Braithwaite S, Verderese C. *Practical Management of Inpatient Hyperglycemia.* Lakeville, CT: Hilliard Publishing; 2005.

Lien LF, Bethel MA, Feinglos MN. In-hospital management of type 2 diabetes mellitus. *Med Clin N Am.* 2004;88(4):1085–1105.

Lien LF, Lane JD. Chapter 29: Pharmacologic factors affecting glycemic control. In: Feinglos MN, Bethel MA, eds. *Contemporary endocrinology: type 2 diabetes mellitus: an evidence-based approach to practical management.* Totowa, NJ: Humana Press; 2008.

Moghissi E, Korytkowski M, DiNardo M, et al. American Association of Clinical Endocrinologists and American Diabetes Association consensus statement on inpatient glycemic control. *Endocr Pract.* 2009;15(4):353–369.

Umpierrez GE, Palacio A, Smiley D. Sliding scale insulin use: myth or insanity? *Am J Med.* 2007;120(7):563–567.

Subject Index

Note: The letters 't' and 'f' followed by the locators represents 'tables' and 'figures' respectively.

A

AADE7™ self-care behaviors
  being active, 44
  glucose monitoring, 45
  healthy coping, 45
  healthy eating, 44
  medications, 45
  problem solving, 45
  reducing risks, 45
Abnormal glucose measurements, 122–129
Acidosis, 22, 51–52, 54 55, 57, 60,
    78t, 81t, 82
Active insulin time, 68
ADA, *see* American Diabetes Association
    (ADA)
Adult Treatment Panel (ATP), 37, 83–84
AG, *see* Anion gap (AG)
All or none approach, 106
α (alpha)-glucosidase inhibitor
  acarbose (precose®)
    inpatient considerations, 85
    mechanism and efficacy, 85
    safety, 85
American Diabetes Association (ADA), 1–2,
    31, 33, 37t, 44, 47, 56, 63, 111, 126
Amylin analog
  pramlintide (symlin®)
    inpatient considerations, 88
    mechanism and efficacy, 87
    safety, 87–88
Analog insulins, 4, 130
  See also Insulin, types, rapid-acting insulin
Anion gap (AG), 22, 36, 54–56, 59–60, 126
Antibiotic therapy, 71
Aspart (Novolog®), 4t–5t, 13, 22–23, 67, 96,
    104t, 105, 108, 122, 129t, 130
ATP, *see* Adult Treatment Panel (ATP)
Autoantibody

categories of, 35
markers, 30t, 35
zinc transporter antibody ZnT8, 35

B

Basal-bolus insulin
  correctional insulin scale, 8
  for patients with type 1/type 2 diabetes, 7
Basal-bolus insulin regimen, 8, 12–13,
    105, 110
Basal dose calculation, 14, 24–25, 73
Basal insulin, 6–8, 13–14, 19, 23–25, 67, 95,
    118, 122, 127, 131–134
Basal rate, 67, 69, 71, 73
Bedside glucose monitoring, 18
Biguanides
  metformin (glucophage®/glucophage
      XR®)
    inpatient considerations, 82
    mechanism and efficacy, 81
    safety, 82
Blood glucose monitoring, 20, 46, 48, 69, 94,
    115t–116t, 118
Blood Glucose Test, 47, 107f
BMI, *see* Body mass index (BMI)
Body mass index (BMI), 10
Bolus calculator, 68
Bolus feeding, 115t, 117
Bolus wizard, 69
Bromocriptine mesylate (Cycloset®),
    80t–81t, 88

C

Calorie counting, 64
Carbohydrate counting, 63–66
Carbohydrate serving, 64
Cardiovascular risk assessment
  high-sensitivity C-reactive protein (hsCRP)
    increase in total CRP, 38

L.F. Lien et al. (eds.), *Glycemic Control in the Hospitalized Patient*,
DOI 10.1007/978-1-60761-006-9, © Springer Science+Business Media, LLC 2011

Cardiovascular risk assessment (*cont.*)
    traditional assays, 38
    lipid profile, 37
CDE, *see* Certified Diabetes Educators (CDE)
Celiac disease, 65
Centers for Disease Control and Prevention
        (CDC), 1
Certified Diabetes Educators (CDE), 47, 102
CGM, *see* Continuous glucose monitoring
        (CGM)
Continuous feeding, 115t
Continuous glucose monitoring (CGM), 73–74
Continuous subcutaneous insulin infusion
        (CSII), 64, 67–69, 72–73, 96t, 104t,
        106, 119, 122, 130, 134, 136
Correctional insulin scale, 8, 12, 14–15, 73,
        105, 107, 135
Correction dose insulin, 122, 126–127
Counterregulatory hormones, 52, 58, 91, 94–95
C-peptide, 2t, 30t, 34–35
CSII, *see* Continuous subcutaneous insulin
        infusion (CSII)
CSII continuation, eligible criterias, 68
Cystic fibrosis, 3, 65, 120

D
Dawn phenomenon, 9, 14
DCCT, *see* Diabetes Control and Complication
        Trial (DCCT)
Dental disease, 65
Detemir insulin, 6
Detemir (Levemir®), 4t, 6, 13, 23, 56, 73, 96t,
        104t, 105, 108, 122, 129t
10% dextrose (D10), 93t, 97f, 117–118, 124,
        131, 134
50% dextrose (D50), 93, 93t, 94f, 98,
        121–122, 123f
Diabetes
    education, 41–48, 111
    in labor, 135
    medication, 46, 110, 125–126, 129,
        131–132
    self-care, 42, 67, 111
Diabetes Control and Complication Trial
        (DCCT), 43
Diabetes mellitus, physiology of
    exogenous insulin, types
        intermediate-acting insulin, 5
        long-acting (basal) insulin, 6
        rapid-acting insulin, 4
        regular and NPH insulin, mixture
            of, 5
        short-acting insulin, 5

pathophysiology
    characteristics, 2t
    MODY, 3–4
    type 1 diabetes, 3
    type 2 diabetes, 3
    prevalence
Diabetes Prevention Program (DPP), 43, 87
Diabetic ketoacidosis (DKA), 2t, 3, 7, 14, 17,
        18t, 30t, 36, 46, 51–62, 72, 78t– 80t,
        126, 132, 135
Dipeptidyl peptidase-4 inhibitors
    sitagliptin (januvia®)/saxagliptin
        (onglyza®)
        inpatient considerations, 87
        mechanism and efficacy, 87
        safety, 87
Discharge planning, 45–46, 65
Discharge regimens, 44, 102, 103t–104t
DKA, *see* Diabetic ketoacidosis
        (DKA)
DKA resolution, 56
Dopamine agonist
    bromocriptine mesylate (cycloset®)
        inpatient considerations, 88
        mechanism and efficacy, 88
        safety, 88
DPP, *see* Diabetes Prevention Program
        (DPP)

E
Education constructs, 44
Electrolytes
    bicarbonate, 57–58
    phosphate, 58
    potassium, 57
    sodium, 57
Empathetic listening, 43
Endocrinology consultation
    retrospective study, 119
    situations considered, 119–120
Enteral nutrition, 8, 113, 117–118,
        122, 134
Euglycemic DKA, 55
Exenatide (Byetta®), 79t, 81t, 86, 132

F
Fasting plasma glucose (FPG), 2t, 31
FDA, *see* Food and Drug Administration
        (FDA)
Food and Drug Administration (FDA), 32,
        88, 128
FPG, *see* Fasting plasma glucose (FPG)
Fructosamine, 30t, 33–34

G

Gastroparesis, 65, 80t, 86
GDH-PQQ, *see* Glucose dehydrogenase
    pyrroloquinoline quinone
    (GDH-PQQ)
GFR, *see* Glomerular filtration rate (GFR)
Glargine insulin, 6
Glargine (Lantus®), 4t, 6, 13, 23, 56, 73, 96t,
    104t, 105, 108, 122, 129t, 134
Glimeperide (Amaryl®), 78t
Glipizide (Glucotrol®), 78t, 81t, 83
Glomerular filtration rate (GFR), 10, 12t
Glucagon, 52, 86–87, 91, 93, 98, 108, 122, 136
Glucagon-like peptide-1 analogs
    exenatide (byetta®), liraglutide
      (victoz α®)
      inpatient considerations, 86
      mechanism and efficacy, 86
      safety, 86
Glucometer, 109, 121
Gluconeogenesis, 82, 91
Glucose
    homeostasis, 1, 3, 35
    meters, 29, 32–33, 74, 109–110, 121
    monitoring, 9, 11, 18–20, 45–48, 58, 69,
      73–74, 93t, 94, 96, 98, 105–106,
      115t–116t, 118, 121–122, 124, 135
    plasma, 29–30
    POCT, 32
    sensor, 67–74, 130
    testing device, 109
    urinary, 32–33
Glucose-based tests
    diabetes screening and diagnosis
      plasma glucose-based tests, categories
        of, 31
    plasma glucose
      uses of, 29
    POCT glucose, 32
    urinary glucose, 32–33
Glucose dehydrogenase pyrroloquinoline
    quinone (GDH-PQQ), 32, 128
Glulisine (Apidra®), 4t, 13, 22–23, 67, 96t,
    104t, 105, 108, 122, 129t
Glyburide (Diaâeta®, Micronase®), 78t,
    81t, 83
Glycated proteins
    conditions causing inaccurate A1C
      readings
      anemia, 33–34
      pregnancy, 34
      recent blood transfusion, 33
      splenectomy, 34

    fructosamine, 34
    hemoglobin A_{1C}
      A1C value and average glucose,
        relationship, 33
    insulin, pro-insulin, and C-peptide
      final phase of production, 35
      markers of, 35
      measurement, 35
    point-of-care A1C
      use in office-based setting, 34

H

Hardware malfunction, 133
Heart Protection Study (HPS), 37–38
Hematocrit level, 32, 128
Hemoglobin A_{1C}, 10, 33–34, 45–46, 55, 125
High-Sensitivity C-Reactive Protein (hsCRP),
    30t, 38
HOMA, *see* Homeostatic model
    assessment (HOMA)
Homeostatic model assessment (HOMA), 35
Hospitalized patients with diabetes mellitus
    autoantibody markers, 35
    cardiovascular risk assessment
      high-sensitivity C-Reactive Protein
        (hsCRP), 38
      lipid profile, 37–38
    glucose-based tests
      diabetes screening and diagnosis, 31
      plasma glucose, 29–30
      POCT glucose, 32
      urinary glucose, 32–33
    glycated proteins
      conditions causing inaccurate A1C
        readings, 33–34
      fructosamine, 34
      hemoglobin A_{1C}, 33
      point-of-care A1C, 34
    insulin, pro-insulin, and C-peptide, 34–35
    ketones
      serum, 36
      urine, 36
    urine microalbumin, 36–37
HPS, *see* Heart Protection Study (HPS)
HsCRP, *see* High-Sensitivity C-Reactive
    Protein (hsCRP)
Humulin®, 5
Hyperglycemia, 125–126
Hyperglycemia with enteral and parenteral
    nutrition/management
    description, 113–114
      enteral feeding formulas, 114t
    in enteral feeding, 117–118

Hyperglycemia with enteral (*cont.*)
   insulin regimens for enteral feeding,
      115t–116t
   total parenteral nutrition, 118
Hyperglycemic emergencies
   diabetic ketoacidosis
      case presentation, 51
      clinical presentation and manifestations,
         52–53
      evaluation, 54–55
      laboratory findings, 55
      management, 57–58
      pathogenesis, 52
      precipitants, 53–54
      simplified pathophysiology, 53f
   DKA, 58
   HHS, 62
   hyperosmolar hyperglycemic state
      clinical presentation and
         manifestations, 59
      differential diagnosis, 54
      evaluation, 59–60
      laboratory findings, 60
      management, 60
Hyperosmolar hyperglycemic state (HHS)
   clinical presentation and manifestations, 59
   differential diagnosis, 59
   evaluation, 59–60
   HHS/DKA, differentiation, 58
   laboratory findings, 60
   management
      electrolytes, 61–62
      insulin, 61
      IV fluids, 61
      vigilance, 62
   precipitants, 59
Hyperosmolar nonketotic hyperglycemia
     (HONK/HNKH), 58
   See also Hyperosmolar hyperglycemic
     state (HHS)
Hypoglycemia, 121–124, 136
   prevention of
      appropriate glucose monitoring
         frequency, 96–98
      appropriate glucose targets, 95–96
      appropriate insulin/medication
         dosages, 95
      D10 algorithm, 97f
      Periprocedural insulin management, 96t
   recognition of
      diagnosis, 92
      hypoglycemia unawareness, causes, 92t
      mechanisms, 91–92

      neurogenic/autonomic symptoms, 92
      neuroglycopenic symptoms, 92
      Whipple's triad components, 92
   risk factors, 98
   treatment of
      algorithm, 94f
      rule of 15s, 92
      steps to confirm and treat, 93t
Hypoglycemia unawareness, 9, 11t, 15t, 74,
     80t, 92t, 96, 98, 110, 120
Hyponatremia, 55, 57, 60

I
Ineffective insulin infusion, 133–134
Inpatient diabetes education, 41–48
   content
      AADE7TM self-care behaviors, 44–45
      published recommendations, synthesis
         of, 45–46
   educators
      CDE, nurse, and dietician, 47–48
      physician and other providers, 47
      staff nurse, 47
   self-care education
      factors interfering, 42–44
      need in hospital, 42
   strategies, 44
   training and support for healthcare
      providers, 48
Inpatient diabetes self-management, 91
Insulin
   allergy, 135
   to carbohydrate ratio, 68–69, 73, 134
   drip, 17–26
   pump, 67–74, 104t, 106, 130, 134, 136–137
      malfunctions, 134–137
      See also Insulin pumps and glucose
         sensors
   reactions, 92
   resistance, 1–3, 10, 35, 81–83, 98, 125, 134
   teaching, 102
   types
      intermediate-acting insulin, 5
      long-acting (basal) insulin, 6
      mixture of regular and nph insulin, 5
      rapid-acting insulin, 4, 4t
      short-acting insulin, 4t, 5
   See also IV insulin infusions
Insulin/non-insulin antidiabetic medication,
     77–89, 102, 103t, 122, 125, 129,
     132–133
Insulin pumps and glucose sensors
   appropriate documentation of settings,
      69–70

continuous glucose monitoring, 73–74
CSII continuation, 68
pump site reactions
    allergic reactions, 72
    site infection, 71–72
    transition to subcutaneous insulin,
        72–73
removal procedures, 68–69
troubleshooting
    hyperglycemia, 70
    hypoglycemia, 70–71
Insulin sensitivity factor (ISF), 68–69, 73, 135
ISF, *see* Insulin sensitivity factor (ISF)
IV insulin infusions
    adjusting the rates
        implementation of nomogram, 19
        multiplication factor, 19
        titrated dose according to institution's
            protocol, 20f–21f
    indications, 18t
    scenarios for use, 17
    special scenario, 19–22
    starting
        bedside glucose monitoring, 18
        initial rate calculations, 18t
    transitioning to subcutaneous insulin
        in NPO patient, 22–26
        overlap and subcutaneous insulin
            initiation, 26

K
Ketones
    serum
        measurement of, 36
        production of, 36
        treatment, 36
    urine
        measurement, 36
        primary advantage of, 36
Ketosis, 54, 136

L
LADA, *see* Latent autoimmune diabetes of the
        adult (LADA)
Lantus®, 4t, 6, 13, 23, 56, 73, 96t, 104t, 105,
        108, 122, 129t
Latent autoimmune diabetes of the adult
        (LADA), 3
LDL, *see* Low-density lipoprotein (LDL)
Levemir®, 4t, 6, 13, 23, 56, 73, 96t, 104t, 105,
        108, 122, 129t, 134
Lien-Spratt IV insulin nomogram, 19, 21f
Lipid panel, 30t, 38
Liquid diet, 64

Liraglutide (Victoza®), 78t, 81t, 86
Lispro (Humalog®), 4t, 13, 22–23, 67, 96t,
        104t, 105, 108, 122, 129t, 130
Long-acting insulin, 5, 13–14, 23–24, 56, 73,
        96t, 104t, 105, 107–108, 115t–116t,
        118, 122, 134
Low-density lipoprotein (LDL), 37–38

M
Maturity onset diabetes of the young (MODY),
        3–4, 120
Mealtime dose calculation, 73
Medical nutrition therapy (MNT), 63–66, 110
    carbohydrate serving, 64
    goals, 63
    hospital care
        discharge planning, 65
        nutrition consult, 64
        related comorbidities, assessment,
            64–65
        supervised calorie counting, 64
Medication timing and administration,
        129–133
Meglitinides
    repaglinide (prandin®)/nateglinide
        (starlix®)
        inpatient considerations, 85
        mechanism and efficacy, 84
        safety, 84–85
Metformin (Glucophage®), 78t, 81t
MNT, *see* Medical nutrition therapy (MNT)
MODY, *see* Maturity onset diabetes of the
        young (MODY)
Multidisciplinary teamwork, 46

N
Nateglinide (Starlix®), 79t, 81t, 84, 132
Neutral protamine hagedorn (NPH), 4t, 5,
        13–14, 25–26, 96, 103t–104t, 105,
        110, 115t, 122, 129t, 130
Nocturnal feeding, 115t–116t, 117, 131
Non-insulin antidiabetic medications in
        inpatient setting
    α (alpha)-glucosidase inhibitor
        acarbose (precose®), 85
    amylin analog
        pramlintide (symlin®), 87–88
    biguanides
        metformin (glucophage®/glucophage
            XR®), 81–82
    and cardiovascular health, 88–89
    dipeptidyl peptidase-4 inhibitors
        sitagliptin (januvia®)/saxagliptin
            (onglyza®), 87

Non-insulin antidiabetic medications (*cont.*)
  dopamine agonist
    bromocriptine mesylate (cycloset®),
      88
  glucagon-like peptide-1 analogs
    exenatide (byetta®), liraglutide
      (victozα®), 86
  meglitinides
    repaglinide (prandin®)/nateglinide
      (starlix®), 84–85
  sulfonylureas
    glipizide (glucotrol®)/glimepiride
      (amaryl ®)/glyburide
      (diaßeta®/glynase prestabs
      ®/micronase®), 83–84
  thiazolidinediones
    pioglitazone (actos®)/rosiglitazone
      (avandia®), 82–83
  and toxicities, 81t
Novolin®, 4t–5t, 12–13, 20, 23, 96t, 103, 122,
    129t
NPH, *see* Neutral protamine hagedorn (NPH)
NPH insulin, 5, 13–14, 25–26, 96t, 103t, 105,
    115t, 129
Nutrition counseling, 44, 64–65

O
Off-pump plan, 69, 73
OGTT, *see* Oral glucose tolerance test (OGTT)
Oral glucose tolerance test (OGTT), 2t, 31–32

P
Patient-centered approaches, 43
Pioglitazone (Actos®), 78t, 82–83
Plasma glucose, 2t, 29–32, 54–55, 59, 68, 77,
    84, 86, 93, 121–122, 126–128, 135
Plasma glucose-based tests, categories of
  fasting plasma glucose (FPG), 31
  oral glucose tolerance test (OGTT), 31–32
  random plasma glucose (RPG), 31
Plate method, 65
POCT, *see* Point-of-care glucose test (POCT)
POCT and plasma glucose readings, 127–129
Point-of-care glucose test (POCT), 29, 32, 96,
    121–122, 124–128, 130
Positive urine ketones, 136
Pramlintide (Symlin®), 80t–81t, 87–88
Prandial insulin, 5, 7, 12, 23–25, 88, 95,
    121–122, 122, 124, 131–132, 134
Prediabetes and diabetes, ADA diagnostic
    criteria, 2t
Premixed insulin regimen, 102
Pro-insulin, 30t, 34–35
Pseudohyponatremia, 60

Pump(s)
  self-management orders, 69–70
  site reactions, 71–73
  therapy, 71

R
Random plasma glucose (RPG), 2t, 31
Rapid-acting insulin, 4–5, 13–14, 20, 22–24,
    56, 67, 73, 96t, 102t, 104t, 105–106,
    108, 115t, 122, 127, 130, 133
  See also Insulin
Regular insulin, 5, 13–14, 18, 20, 25–26,
    56, 58, 73, 96t, 103t–104t, 105,
    115t–116t, 117–118, 122, 133–134
Repaglinide (Prandin®), 79t, 81t, 84–85, 132
Rosiglitazone (Avandia®), 79t, 81t
RPG, *see* Random plasma glucose (RPG)
Rule of 15s, 92, 98, 123
Rule of thumb, discharge planning, 65

S
Saxagliptin (Onglyza®), 80t, 81t, 87
Self-care education
  factors interfering
    patient misconceptions, 42
    provider misconceptions, 42
    specific tactics, 42–43
Severe hyperglycemia, 18t, 35, 37, 58, 60,
    126–127, 131
Sitagliptin (Januvia®), 80t, 81t, 87
Sliding scale, 8, 43, 105, 126
Somogyi effect, 9
Split-mix insulin regimen, 13, 105
Subcutaneous insulin
  basal-bolus insulin
    special care situations, 8
  blood glucose targets, 9
  choosing an insulin regimen
    correctional insulin scale, 14–15
    intermediate- and short-acting insulin,
      13–14
    long- and rapid-acting insulin, 13
    for patients taking glucocorticoids, 12
    for patients with renal impairment, 12
    renal impairment modified, 12t
    scenarios and examples, 10–12
    situations modified for insulin dose, 11t
    total daily dose, distribution, 12–13
    total daily insulin dose, calculation, 10
  glucose monitoring
    frequency, 9
  outpatient to inpatient care, transition, 8
Sulfonylureas

glipizide (glucotrol®)/glimepiride (amaryl®)/glyburide (diaßeta®/glynase prestabs®/ micronase®)
  inpatient considerations, 84
  mechanism and efficacy, 83
  safety, 84
Supervised calorie counting, 64

T
Target blood glucose range, 67, 106
Teachable moment, 45, 47
Thiazolidinediones
  pioglitazone (actos®)/rosiglitazone (avandia®)
    hypoglycemia, risk factors, 84t
    inpatient considerations, 83
    mechanism and efficacy, 82–83
    safety, 83
Total daily dose of insulin, 11t, 114
Total Parenteral Nutrition (TPN), 7–8, 13, 72, 116t, 118, 122
Total plasma osmolality, 55
TPN, *see* Total parenteral nutrition (TPN)
Transitioning to outpatient care
  behavior recommendations, 110
  checklist for discharge, 102f
  choice of discharge regimen, 102–105
    basal-bolus insulin regimen, 105
    premixed insulin regimen, 102
    split-mix insulin regimen, 105
  follow-up appointments, 110–111

glucose monitoring post-discharge and reporting results, 105–106
hypo- and hyperglycemia, 106
  sample discharge instructions, 107f
insulin teaching, 102
medication regimen, 101–102
prescriptions, 106–110
  sample prescriptions, 109f
recording and reporting, 106
sample discharge instructions, 111
target glucose ranges, 106
Troubleshooting, 70–71
Tube feeding, 97, 113, 115t, 133–134
Type 1 diabetes, 2t, 3, 7–8, 10–11, 14, 19, 30t, 35, 46, 51, 65, 67, 78t–80t, 87, 91, 103t, 110, 117, 119, 125, 131, 135
Type 2 diabetes, 2t, 3, 7, 10–11, 31–32, 35, 37–38, 58, 67, 77, 80t, 88, 103t, 117, 125, 135–136

U
U-500 insulin, 133
Urine microalbumin, 30, 36–37, 45
  other possible causes, 37
    identification, 37

W
Water deficit, 56
Whipple's triad components, 92, 98

Z
Zinc transporter antibody ZnT8, 35